ADVANCE PRAISE FOR *LIVING LONG & LOVING IT*

"This gem of a book brings together scientific principles of aging, osteopathy, physiology, and health psychology, along with the author's personal narrative on aging well. Rather than the traditional medical focus on how to 'prevent disease,' Korr speaks to how we can 'seek health' and offers basic strategies that the reader can undertake to identify potential barriers to well-being, and ways to overcome these challenges to create healthful aging. He succeeds without preaching, and will surely convince anyone who picks up this refreshing book.... It will encourage even the most ardent couch potato to get up, get moving, and to make the choice for health as a way of life."

—Sue Levkoff, ScD, associate professor of psychiatry,
Brigham and Women's Hospital,
a Harvard Medical School teaching affiliate,
and editor of *Ageing International*

"... offers a first-hand account of the habits and practices that helped to foster Dr. Korr's long, happy, and productive life. The authors support their conclusions by describing and referencing a large body of scientific studies. As a physician who treats patients with chronic rheumatic diseases, I believe that this book can serve as an important reference for patients to help them manage their lives as well as their disease."

—Arthur M. Bobrove, MD, Department of Internal Medicine,
Division of Rheumatology, Palo Alto Medical Foundation,
and clinical professor of medicine (adjunct),
Stanford University Medical School

"... a readable and engaging guide to discovering 'the capacity of the self-healing physician within.' ... [The authors] employ the principles of osteopathy, celebrating the oneness of the body as an integrated community of mutual influence where one part affects the others, where body and mind are interdependent and are one; they do this not in some arcane or unapproachable manner but rather in a way that is readily understandable and, quite frankly, inspirational. The result is a book for adults of any age who wish to understand not only their health but also themselves. It is informative without being preachy, profound in a way that becomes apparent midway through reading. Aging well is a consequence."

—Edward F. Ansello, PhD,
a fellow of the Gerontological Society of America
and director of the Virginia Center on Aging

"In reading and critiquing this book, I found it extremely interesting and, based on past experiences, continue to appreciate Dr. Irvin Korr's philosophy and passion for life."

—Richard G. Stefanacci, DO, FACOS,
geriatrician and medical director,
Forest Hill Healthcare Center, New Jersey

LIVING LONG
& LOVING IT

Irvin M. Korr, PʜD, &
Rene J. McGovern, PʜD

LIVING LONG
& LOVING IT

Achieving a HEALTHY
and ACTIVE Lifestyle

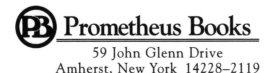

Prometheus Books

59 John Glenn Drive
Amherst, New York 14228–2119

Published 2008 by Prometheus Books

Inquiries should be addressed to
Prometheus Books
59 John Glenn Drive
Amherst, New York 14228–2119
VOICE: 716–691–0133, ext. 210
FAX: 716–691–0137
WWW.PROMETHEUSBOOKS.COM

12 11 10 09 08   5 4 3 2 1

Library of Congress Cataloging-in-Publication Data

Korr, Irvin M.
    Living long and loving it : achieving a healthy and active lifestyle / by Irvin M. Korr and Rene J. McGovern. — 1st American pbk. ed.
       p. cm.
    Includes bibliographical references and index.
    ISBN 978–1–59102–572–6
    1. Longevity. 2. Health. I. McGovern, Rene J. II. Title.

RA776.75.K67 2008
613.2—dc22

                                          2007051809

CONTENTS

PART 5   REINFORCEMENT OF LESSONS LEARNED

FOREWORD
Janet Meneley Korr

It is very gratifying to see this, my husband's last book, published. He began writing it the year following his retirement from the University of North Texas Health Science Center in Fort Worth, Texas, in his eightieth year. At that time, he claimed to have been the oldest state employee in Texas. That claim speaks to the essence of this book and to his great vitality into his late years.

This book is really a distillation of his professional and personal knowledge and life experiences. He believed deeply in what he wrote and carried its practice into all of his late years. He would be pleased and honored to know that it has, at last, come into print.

I would like to acknowledge and express my deepest gratitude to Rene J. McGovern, PhD, at A. T. Still University–Kirksville College of Osteopathic Medicine, and Jason Haxton, director of the Still National Osteopathic Museum.

FOREWORD
David Korr

My father's sense of humor was legendary. He loved a good joke, from the subtlest to the silliest, and especially enjoyed puns and parodies. Among his writings are some pseudomedical papers describing imaginary illnesses, such as "nephrotrichosis"—hairy kidneys.

Growing up, I enjoyed my father's playful side, but I learned that when *genuine* issues of health were the subject, he was not inclined to joke. He regarded the best possible health as one's profound, lifelong responsibility and not—as it is for so many—simply a matter of casual attention and routine maintenance. Guided by his own research and the teachings of osteopathy, he considered us all beneficiaries of bodies (and minds) that, through natural mechanisms, seek balance, stability, ease, and harmony. Honoring nature's gift to us by nourishing it and freeing it to work for us was, he believed, part of the very meaning of a life lived well.

Indeed, over the years, his counsel to me regarding various follies or excesses was as likely to be about their effects on my health as about other, perhaps more obvious, issues. I've never forgotten his description of the physiological effects of useless anger. (We shared the failing of a short temper—a problem he discusses in these pages.) Above all, though, it was his own unending quest for self-understanding and for a healthful engagement with the challenges and rewards of life that served as a model for me, as it still does.

PREFACE

"This book has been written for those, regardless of age, who are motivated to achieve levels of health that will enable them to enjoy a long and active life. I hope that it will also influence some who, by virtue of their roles in society, have the responsibility and the power to support such efforts and to remove economic, educational, and environmental obstacles."

—Irvin M. Korr, 1997

A t no time in the past has healthy aging been more critical. With the demographics of aging descending upon us and the federal deficit looming, healthcare resources are becoming scarcer for those who cannot afford them. Medical education has been trying to gear up for the impending storm, but it may not be enough.

Years ago in a tiny village in the Midwest, a physician and son of an itinerant minister began searching for the sources of good health. It is with that man's legacy that Irvin "Kim" Korr discovered a secret to aging well. It was his intention to share that secret with the world in this book.

Kim Korr was trained as a physiologist at Princeton University at a time when a doctoral degree was the purview of only the extremely bright and privileged. Dr. Korr was both. After securing an academic position at New York University, the influence of World War II and the communist threat sent Dr. Korr to a little town in the Midwest (Kirksville, Missouri) to "find out what was going on there." The secret to aging well that he found there was osteopathy, and it would change Dr. Korr's life forever. His hope, before he died, was that this book will do the same for you.

I met Kim Korr only once, in 1998 at the Broadmoor Hotel in Colorado Springs during the annual meeting of the American Academy of Osteopathy (AAO). He was eighty-nine years old and had the youthful vigor I had come to expect from people in the osteopathic profession.

Let me explain. During my first visit to Kirksville, when my husband had his final interview before becoming president of the Kirksville College of Osteopathic Medicine (or KCOM, the founding college of osteopathic medicine), I saw there was something special about the people who lived there. They had a youthful vitality, a sparkle in their eyes, and pep in their even gait. I did not really know what osteopathic medicine was at that time, but I remember saying to myself that my husband and I would grow old well if we chose to move there. We did choose to move, said good-bye to our life in the city, and left Case Western Reserve University for Kirksville in 1997.

It was in 1998, as I was beginning a qualitative research study comparing doctors of osteopathy (DOs) and allopathic physicians (MDs), that my husband and I went to our first academy meeting. It just so happened that Dr. Korr was giving a keynote address at the meeting, and we were scheduled to have lunch with him and his wife, Jan, after the talk. I had already heard of his reputation as a rigorous researcher ("the best the field had known") and as an exacting professor of physiology. Many a KCOM alumni had talked about struggling with his course but said so with great respect. I was excited to be meeting one of the many legends of the osteopathic profession. When we traveled to state conventions, we frequently heard stories that featured Kim Korr, Max Gutensohn, and Duke Snider. I had come to know those names well.

Nearly eight years after our memorable three-hour lunch with Kim and Jan Korr, the head of the Still National Osteopathic Museum, Jason Haxton, called me with a request to complete a manuscript on healthy aging by Dr. Korr that had been found in the archives. My mind went back in time to our afternoon together and to the great respect that DOs had for Dr. Korr's research. In addition, since our meeting in 1998, my knowledge and training in aging as well as my immersion in osteopathic research and philosophy had expanded. Therefore, I was excited on both an intellectual and a personal level about completing the manuscript. I was also honored that Jan Korr would entrust the manuscript to me.

My contribution to this book has been threefold. First, along with help from A. T. Still University and the Still National Osteopathic Museum, we converted the manuscript from the archives into a living document. Dr. Korr began this book in the 1980s. The copy we had needed to be put into electronic format and updated. Luckily, Dr. Korr's concepts were ahead of his time. His research had always been cutting edge, and he did not limit his thinking. Second, I needed to couch his ideas within the extensive work on aging that had been done since he put the manuscript to rest in the 1990s. Finally, I worked to assure that the voice you hear will be Dr. Korr's throughout this book as he tells his story of healthful aging. He apologizes frequently, not wanting to appear less than humble. He is a teacher par excellence. Through the interweaving of his story with his ideas, he teaches profound principles for health as well as provides physiological and neurophysiological knowledge that will change how you think and behave.

After working with this manuscript for two years, I feel as if I have been tutored by one of the best teachers of the twentieth century. As much as I believed that I understood my own fields of aging and of health psychology, Dr. Korr's synthesis of his own research and application to the laboratory of his own life made some of the messiness of my own understanding elegantly clear. I invite you to allow this master teacher to mentor you, and I hope you embrace this book.

Dr. Korr has interwoven four themes. Primarily, the book serves as a guide on how to achieve successful aging. As a physiologist, an award-winning medical educator, and a respected scientist, Dr. Korr has illustrated key principles by utilizing his personal experiences to make them meaningful and easily understood. The foundation of his insights and his life transformation are based on an integration of the principles of osteopathy developed by A. T. Still and the training in physiology Dr. Korr received at Princeton University. Well versed in the knowledge of his time, Dr. Korr immersed himself in osteopathy and was transformed by it. His research on the principles of osteopathy was ahead of its time and has been supported by current research in psychoneuroimmunology. It is both his fundamental knowledge and the process of transformation that Dr. Korr wished to share with the world as his legacy before he died. Unfortunately, Dr. Korr died at the age of ninety-four and was unable to complete this project. Therefore, it is my great privilege to act as midwife to his legacy, along with his widow, Jan Korr.

Dr. Korr hoped to impart other key themes regarding his personal transformation through osteopathy. He had a deep understanding of the evolutional influences of biology; the capacity of the self-healing physician within; the unity of the body, mind, and spirit; the notion of commitment and personal responsibility in achieving and maintaining health; and the value of osteopathic treatments and other types of musculoskeletal activity. At times, he plays down osteopathy because he did not want to preach, but throughout the book one can see its influence on his life-changing journey. I will include in the epilogue a brief history of osteopathy, a brief review of the current status of evidence for osteopathic manipulative therapy, and a further integration of Dr. Korr's ideas in my field of aging and health psychology. I will also offer additional resources for those who would like more in-depth knowledge, and I will share how one might find an osteopath in both the United States and most other countries of the world. I hesitate to say more lest I prevent you from meeting the real author and beginning your life-changing journey toward healthy aging.

Rene J. McGovern, MA, MS, PhD, OblSB

INTRODUCTION

"Health is the best defense against disease."
—I. M. Korr

T his book has been written for those, regardless of age, who are motivated to achieve levels of health that will enable them to enjoy a long and active life. I hope that it will also influence some who, by virtue of their roles in society, have the responsibility and the power to support such efforts and to remove economic, educational, and environmental obstacles.

What is offered in this book is soundly based in science, but it is not intended to be a scientific textbook. However, for those who wish to delve more deeply into the scientific documentation and explanations, references have been provided in the text to appropriate appendices and publications.

Nineteenth-century British poet Robert Browning stated in his poem "Rabbi Ben Ezra" that we should "Grow old along with me! / The best is yet to be, / The last of life, for which the first was made."[1] This book is intended as an affirmation that the last part of one's life can indeed be the best part of life. The opportunity is open to each of us to make it so. It is true that a healthy, vigorous, fulfilling old age and long life are the natural culmination of healthy living. Once we understand what is meant by healthy living, it is never too early, or too late, to start along the path toward better health. Therefore, my purpose is to offer an understanding of the principles that I have found to be reliable guides to living healthfully and aging successfully.

My understanding of healthy living comes, in part, from more than a half century of experience as a physiologist, medical educator, and researcher. Equally important, what I offer is the product of my personal experience in the past forty-plus years during which I learned these healthy-living concepts and put them into daily practice. They have enabled me, into my nineties, to enjoy youthful health and vigor as well as all the good things that they make possible. I would like to stress that these healthy-living concepts are solidly based in human biology and are the very foundations of health. I hope that you, too, may adopt them, in your own way, as a means to a longer, richer life.

I would like to begin your journey toward better health with questions. In my many years of teaching, I have discovered that people learn best when learning is preceded by questions specifically formulated to elicit answers within the students' own minds. Unfortunately, many teachers, especially those more concerned with what is taught rather than with what is learned, are inclined to burden their students' minds with thousands of answers to unasked questions. For want of mental hooks, the answers either remain unabsorbed or soon drift out of memory. To avoid that pedagogical sin, I would like to suggest several provocative questions for you to ask yourself as you prepare to seek answers.

My first question is probably one of the most frequently asked and, at the same time, one of the least frequently answered: "How are you?" Before you answer, please think carefully. Instead of giving one of the conventional reflex responses, such as "I'm fine, thank you," imagine that you are answering a close and caring friend, who will reject your perfunctory response with, "No, I mean how are you, *really?*"

Well, how are you really? Would you say that your health is excellent, good, fair, or poor? How did you arrive at that assessment and by what criteria? How do you appraise the health of others? If you would like to be healthier, what precisely do you mean by that? Is it not being sick, or is there more to it than that? How would you go about becoming healthier? How would you know whether you are making progress and when you have reached your goal? Do you think it is possible to have one or more diseases and still experience well-being?

How do you feel about getting older? How do you feel about getting old? Very old? How do you envision yourself as an aged person? What do you see as healthy aging and healthy old age? Can one be healthy though old? Since the older we get, the closer we are to death, isn't aging itself a pathological process? Therefore, is healthy aging really extended living or just prolonged dying? Is having remained healthy in old age the same as having remained young?

If you are already a senior or very senior citizen, are you satisfied with the state of your health? What, realistically, would you like to improve? What would it take on your part to bring about that improvement? Are you willing to do, or stop doing, whatever is necessary to achieve improvement?

As you prepare to read this book, you will find the reading more profitable if you reflect a while on such questions as those suggested above as well as any others that may occur to you. By doing so, you will enhance your personal meaning and pleasure as you journey toward healthier living.

The first chapter is a personal saga—mine. I begin that way because as I reviewed my health history from my viewpoint as a scientist, I gained some clarity about health and how to have it, and about the achievement of a healthy, active, and happy old age. I have been encouraged to share the resulting insights more widely by the grateful responses of numerous audiences with whom I have shared them in the past few years. I hope that you, too, will find them enlightening.

NOTE

1. R. Browning, "Rabbi Ben Ezra," in *Robert Browning*, ed. A. Roberts (Oxford: Oxford University Press, 1997).

PART 1

METAMORPHOSIS

"My earlier fear of death—could it have been a disguised fear of life?"

—I. M. Korr

Chapter 1

WHAT IS YOUR SECRET?

"Having spent most of my life seeking, being given, and discovering countless and diverse answers, only recently have I begun to discover life's most fruitful questions."

—I. M. Korr

During the past twenty-five years or so, I learned to expect a surprised response from persons who had just discovered my age: "You sure don't look—or act—that old. What's your secret?" For most of those years, I received the question as an implied compliment, to which I usually responded in feigned modesty with some flippant acknowledgment that turned off further inquiry.

As I passed into my middle and then late seventies, the question "What is your secret?" became more frequent and insistent. Clearly, people really wanted to know how a person as old as I could appear to be so much more youthful than they thought could (or should) be expected. What, they wanted to know, accounted for the phenomenon of a person born in 1909 who had remained unbent, flat-bellied, agile, and vigorous and was still fully engaged professionally, with continually widening interests; who was still athletically active; and who was still living as enthusiastically as in any previous period, and perhaps even more so.

FAMILY HISTORY

What, then, is the secret of my good fortune? It is certainly not evident in my family history. As a small child, I was aware of the frailty of my father, who, in my fifth or sixth year, was sent away to a tuberculosis sanatorium for a year following a nearly fatal hemorrhage of the lungs. Throughout the rest of his short life, he suffered from impaired circulation in the legs, which made walking difficult and painful. He was also the victim of assorted allergies and recurrent infections. My father died in early middle age of coronary thrombosis, as had both of his parents. As I write this, I am saddened that I have no memory of his having played with me as a child or of my paternal grandparents, who died in my first year of life.

While the maternal side of my family was blessed with longer, less impaired lives, nevertheless, hypertension and hyperthyroidism were chronic problems for my mother, her mother, and her brother; in addition, there were breast tumors, one fatal brain tumor, and two deaths due to congestive heart failure.

MY FIRST FORTY YEARS

Until I left my family home at age twenty-three to complete my graduate studies at Princeton University, physical complaints and chronic illness were so much a part of my daily environment that I grew up with the unconscious conviction that ill health and early death by heart attack were also my destiny. Every skipped heartbeat, palpitation, or stitch in the rib cage reinforced that expectation. Athletic activity, toward which I already felt little inclination, was easily shunned for being hazardous to my survival. I lived cautiously and conservatively, avoiding unnecessary exertion, in order to save my energies for necessary tasks. No wonder I was dubbed a precocious hypochondriac!

I recall an incident in my twenty-fifth year when I found myself jubilantly dashing up the stairs of the university biology building to announce to fellow graduate students that I had just passed my final oral examination for the PhD degree. I halted in midflight, reminding myself that I was no longer as young as I used to be and that the beginning of my professional career was no time to precipitate a heart attack. I completed the climb to the third floor at a stately life-preserving pace.

Upon completing my work for the doctorate and an additional year as postdoctoral fellow, I joined the faculty of the New York University School of Medicine in 1936. In 1942, I took a leave of absence to conduct research for the War Department until the war's end in 1945. Then aged thirty-six, I viewed myself as middle-aged and headed for the inevitable decline. I continued to live my cautious life, reserving my energy for my work and my family in the hope of gaining some additional time. In the fall of 1945, I accepted an appointment as professor and chairman of the Department of Physiology at the Kirksville College of Osteopathy and Surgery (currently Kirksville College of Osteopathic Medicine, a part of A. T. Still University) in Kirksville, Missouri. (The founding of the college in 1892 marks the founding of osteopathy as a reform movement in medicine. Today, there are twenty-six colleges of osteopathic medicine.) I intended to stay only a year, but what I found there was so challenging that I soon made a long-term commitment. I remained until my (first) retirement thirty years later.

What I found so challenging and exciting at my new position were perspectives of health and disease that I had not previously encountered, either as a patient or as a member of a medical faculty. I found myself puzzled and intellectually challenged by the emphasis on the care of the total person and not merely the affected organ, function, or symptom; on the body's own healing power; on the partnership of patient and physician in nurturing that power; and on the role of the musculoskeletal system in health and disease.

It was not, however, until five years later, when I was forty-one years old, that these perspectives began to have personal as well as academic meaning for me and that my lifelong assumptions about my own health and early demise were challenged for the very first time.

THE BEGINNING OF THE SECOND FORTY-YEAR PERIOD

One morning in the fall of 1950, as I ended a physiology lecture, I was approached at the podium by a recently appointed faculty physician. He introduced himself as Dr. John Chace and, without preliminaries, offered me his clinical services. (At that time, fees were not an issue since free healthcare in the clinics and hospital of the college was available to all faculty and staff.)

Startled by his proposal, I asked, "Why? I'm not sick."

"No," he responded, "you may not be sick yet with a namable disease, but you're not very well either!"

What a startling idea! While observing and listening to physicians for many years, both as a patient and colleague, I had unquestioningly accepted the conventional premise, unarticulated but eloquently expressed in practice, that everyone is in either of two states: we are either sick or well. Further, only the sick are eligible for healthcare since the well have nothing to cure. Not only had the phrase "not very well" implied to me a concept of gradations or degrees of health, but Dr. Chace was, in effect, offering me an option I did not know I had. He was offering me the chance to *upgrade* my health.

I asked what had led him to such an unfavorable assessment of my health. He imitated perfectly my habit of leaning on the lectern throughout my lectures. He described my labored breathing, shoulders visibly rising and falling with each breath; my frequent sighing; the gradual fading of my voice and the change in my pallor; and the resulting collapse into my office chair after each lecture.

"Of course," I protested. "I pour a lot of energy into my lectures."

"Not that much," he said with a faint smile.

Entirely on the basis of his observations of my posture and the way I moved, he was even able to describe in detail my severe right-sided headaches and backaches. By way of explanation, he pointed to the almost fixed tilt of my head to the right, due to contracted muscles, and the compensatory curve in the lower back that brought my eyes level.

How could I not be impressed by his observations and by their interpretation? I accepted, with some uncertainty, Dr. Chace's caring offer. After all, what did I have to lose?

My first, and longest, visit to Dr. Chace's office was devoted entirely to a physical examination performed, not only by himself, but by internists on the clinical staff as well as x-ray and lab technicians. In addition to diagnostic procedures in common use in those days, Dr. Chace performed a palpatory survey of my entire body with his hands, assessing muscular tensions and tissue textures in every area, prodding for sites of tenderness that he seemed to locate with remarkable precision, and testing for ease and range of motion of virtually every joint in my body.

THE RIGID BODY AND THE TREATMENT

He found, as he had expected based on my gait and posture, that I was physically as inflexible as a much older man. He was especially concerned about two areas, my neck and chest. My neck was a problem because the rigid tilt of my head, aside from causing headaches, demanded compensatory adjustments elsewhere in my body. My chest was a concern because what he found there seriously impaired my respiration, so vital to general health. While each rib hinges on the spine and should be freely mobile, mine had become nearly immobilized by stiffness in those joints. In addition, he could find little evidence that I was using my diaphragm during respiration. As a consequence, Dr. Chace said my chest had to be lifted and dropped with each breath, "like an orange crate," instead of having the ribs alternately drawing apart and together, "like the folds in an accordion." For me, the simple act of breathing had become so labored and inefficient, and my lungs were so poorly ventilated, that these two reasons alone could account for my lagging energies.

Dr. Chace and I agreed that I would make weekly visits to the clinic. During each thirty-minute visit, Dr. Chace would apply manipulative procedures designed to gradually restore freedom of motion in every part of my musculoskeletal system, including the neck and rib cage. During the first few visits, he also introduced me to the concept of personal responsibility for my health by teaching me additional exercises to be done at home as a way to augment and sustain the therapeutic effects of the treatments. These included stretching and bending exercises for flexibility and abdominal breathing exercises to enhance my diaphragm's respiratory role. The frequency of my treatment sessions would be reduced as we made progress, but he prepared me to expect that treatments would need to continue for some time. My own responsibility for my health would continue for the rest of my life. (See the sidebar on p. 30 for an explanation of the stated objectives, effects, and essential principles of osteopathic manipulative treatment.)

THE BODILY TRANSFORMATION

As the course of treatments continued, first at weekly and then monthly intervals, and as ease of motion improved, I found myself enjoying moving for the first time. I began to walk between my home and the college, a round trip of three miles, and often twice a day when I returned to the lab in the evening or had lunch at home. A nightly walk with the family dog also became part of my newly pleasurable routine.

I recall two evening walks with special poignancy. The first came after only a few weeks of treatment and home exercises when my neck had become more flexible and more nearly erect. As I walked, I discovered with some alarm that the positioning of my head was no longer automatic! I found myself consciously trying to align my eyes with horizontal structures in my line of vision. Apparently the reflexes that controlled the orientation of my head had been so long attuned to the tilt as the neutral position that they couldn't take over until they were appropriately reset. As I recall, it was not until the following evening that I could, with some confidence, delegate responsibility once again to my reflexes.

The second incident came a few weeks later on another evening walk. I had been walking more briskly than usual and felt the need to take a deeper breath. As I was experiencing none of the accustomed resistance, I took what must have been the very first full breath of my entire life. Aside from the momentary pain as parts of my lungs opened and filled in unaccustomed ways, the immediate emotional release was unexpected and enormous. I leaned against a tree and sobbed with total abandon for what seemed a long time, then I walked home in utter peace. I believe I have been breathing slowly, deeply, and easily from that moment on. In retrospect, this was the beginning of a continuing transformation, both mental and physical.

Shortly after, my walking became brisker and longer. Then, the impulse came to break into a run during my evening walks just because it felt good. Running alternately with walking became a part of my daily pleasure. After taking up jogging (which in those days was still an unfamiliar term and activity), I asked Dr. Chace, who was an accomplished athlete, why he had never suggested exercise, other than the flexibility exercises, to me. His answer was simple: "In order for there to be motion, there must be *freedom* of motion. I knew that you would respond when you were ready." Having become much freer, motion had indeed come spontaneously and easily, bringing with it much pleasure and other welcome changes.

With my growing ease of motion came unprecedented body awareness. I seemed to sense what was good for me and what was not. With my wife's eager cooperation and the recommendations of my clinical colleagues, we changed to a much more healthy diet. Having unconsciously made a commitment to my health, I also gave up tobacco after many years of pipe smoking.

MANIPULATIVE THERAPY

The following explanation of manipulative therapy has been directly excerpted from a book I edited, *The Neurobiologic Mechanisms in Manipulative Therapy*.

What Is Manipulative Therapy?

Manipulative therapy involves the application of accurately determined and specifically directed manual forces to the body. Its objective is to improve mobility in areas that are restricted, whether the restrictions are within joints, in connective tissues, or in skeletal muscles. The consequences may be the improvement of posture and locomotion, the relief of pain and discomfort, the improvement of function elsewhere in the body, and enhancement of the sense of well-being.

Diagnosis, leading to the selection of body sites for manipulation and the mode of manipulation, is based on analysis of the patient's history and complaints and on the evaluation of signs provided by palpation (tissue texture, muscular and fascial [connective tissue] tension, joint motion and compliance, skin temperature and moisture), by visual observation (body contour, posture, locomotion, skin color), and by radiographic and other instrumental means.

Manipulative procedures, even in the hands of the same practitioner, vary according to the findings and their changes in each visit; they vary from practitioner to practitioner, from patient to patient, and, for the same patient, from visit to visit. Manipulative therapy is no more a uniform therapeutic entity than is surgery, psychiatry, or pharmacotherapeutics. Clinical effects are thought to be achieved through improvement in musculoskeletal biomechanics, in dynamics of the body fluids (including blood circulation and lymphatic drainage), and in nervous function.*

---

*I. M. Korr, ed., *The Neurobiologic Mechanisms in Manipulative Therapy* (New York: Plenum, 1978), pp. xv–xvi.

INTRODUCTION TO A NEW WAY OF LIFE

No less important and perhaps, in the long run, even more important than Dr. Chace's skilled treatments were his patient explanations of the concepts that guided osteopathic practice. By relating those principles to my own care, he taught them to me in a deeply personal manner. This, in turn, led me to begin an independent and deeper study of the concepts. I found their origins in ancient history and in many cultures.[1]

Through research and study, I investigated the body structure and processes that underlie the principles as well as the ways to apply them to improve my own health and that of my family. I found the principles not only scientifically sound, as I shall explain, but also poetically beautiful.

Thanks to my fascination with this new (for me) philosophy, our course in physiology at the medical college was also transformed. I became aware, as director of the course, that it no longer sufficed to teach how the average heart, for example, functioned. It was our obligation as teachers of physicians-to-be to also teach the ways in which each organ and organ system served the person and how the quality of function was influenced by the kind of person and the kind of life. We therefore sought to teach physiology in the context of human life, human diversity, and human frailty.

TRANSFORMATION OF THE PERSON

I adopted the osteopathic philosophy, a new yet ancient way of interpreting natural law, as a way of life. This commitment hastened and deepened the transformation that had begun at the physical level and started to influence other aspects of my being. Flexibility of body seemed to invite and facilitate a comparable, and welcome, flexibility and openness of mind. With my newfound energies, my interests and activities began to rapidly extend beyond home, the classroom, and the laboratory and into the community. I delved into areas outside my own discipline, such as other sciences, the arts, and the humanities.

I found in myself not only a new, nonjudgmental tolerance but also an appreciation and a love of my colleagues and my students. Anger and resentments seemed to dissolve. I became a more relaxed and effective teacher, researcher, and scholar. My life became a continual quest for new challenges of body and mind as well as new opportunities for growth. At the age of forty-six, I earned a private pilot's license to fly single-engine aircraft. At the age of fifty, I took up tennis. I enjoy participating in a variety of sports, to which I added cross-country skiing following a move to Colorado.

As my health and outlook improved, changes in attitude toward my work also occurred quite spontaneously. Having always lived and worked with a sense of urgency, I became aware at some point in my sixties that I was living with a pervading feeling of timelessness and unhurriedness. My work, like my leisure, had become a source of gratification rather than a compulsion or a drive for recognition. Happily, I continued to live with the disquieting and tantalizing feeling that I still "don't know what I want to be when I grow up" as though some work opportunity is waiting for me that will be even more fulfilling. At the age of eighty-four, I became aware that the quest had changed to "What is the best use of me at this stage of my life?" I explored a variety of alternatives.

I continued in medical education until 1989 when, at the age of eighty, I retired as professor emeritus from the North Texas College of Osteopathic Medicine in Fort Worth, Texas. I remained fully engaged, however, as an author, a visiting lecturer, and a participant in professional conferences in the United States and abroad, in organizational work, and in a variety of volunteer services in my community.

An amusing incident during a very tragic time in my life eloquently symbolizes my transformation. In my late sixties and soon after the death of my first wife, I found myself burdened with the premiums of four unnecessary life insurance policies. I had taken them out almost thirty years earlier in anticipation of an early death and several years before discovering that I could have happier options if I assumed responsibility for my health. I asked a local agent to advise me regarding the appropriate disposition of the policies.

On examining them, he said with a hint of a smile, "Gee, Doctor, that's too bad."

"What's too bad?" I asked.

"You obviously bet on an early death," he responded, "and you lost."

THE SECRET

What, then, is the secret of my good fortune? What are the factors responsible for my new joy of living and the forgotten expectation of illness and early death? Almost certainly, the factor that initiated the change was the enormous improvement of bodily flexibility, the freedom of motion (and of breath) that I experienced as a result of my osteopathic treatments with Dr. Chace. I am convinced, however, that the sustaining factors have been (1) my deliberate commitment to health, (2) assuming personal responsibility for my health in conjunction with osteopathic care, and (3) applying my elaborations of the new principles to my life. I learned that these principles were much more than a guide to clinical practice. I found them to be a valuable guide to the teaching of medical physiology. They also raised new kinds of questions for research. In addition, I discovered that the same principles could be a guide to healthful and joyful living.

I chose to adopt these principles as my way of life and, subsequently, learned that health is a way of life. While these principles are identified here as osteopathic principles, their roots are in antiquity and in many cultures.[2] It is to the credit of A. T. Still, the founder of the osteopathic medical profession, that he adopted and enriched these tenets.[3] Further, the osteopathic profession continues to develop highly effective methods for implementing them. It has based a system of practice upon these principles that also incorporates all of modern medical technology. In addition, osteopathic physicians continue to test and develop osteopathic principles through research.[4]

While the origin of these principles was entirely empirical, they are the synthesis of clinical experience and observation extending over centuries.[5] Beginning in 1945, my research in the laboratory and in the library has been devoted to seeking knowledge and understanding of the biological processes and mechanisms in the human being that account for these clinical experiences and observations.[6] As a result, both I and the professional readers of my research publications have a growing comprehension of the scientific foundations of osteopathic principles.

Having lived by those same osteopathic tenets for over forty years and richly profited from that long experience, I have learned that they compose a healthful way of thinking, behaving, being, and becoming. Others who have made a commitment to their health and assumed responsibility for it have found these guiding principles as rewarding and as transforming as I have, even when adopted late in life. So that you, too, may have the opportunity to live joyfully in the later years of your life, I intend to offer my personal interpretations and elaborations of these guiding principles in part 2. In part 3, I will attempt to dismantle unnecessary barriers and challenge the origins of human vulnerability. Finally, in part 4, I will walk you through ways of creating your own well-being until you, too, break into a run along the path of wellness and healthful aging.

NOTES

1. J. J. McGovern and R. J. McGovern, *Your Healer Within: A Unified Field Theory of Healthcare* (Tucson, AZ: Fenestra, 2003).

2. Ibid.

3. A. T. Still, *Osteopathy, Research and Practice* (1910; repr., Seattle: Eastland Press, 1992).

4. G. J. D. Bergman et al., "Manipulative Therapy in Addition to Usual Medical Care for Patients with Shoulder Dysfunction and Pain," *Annals of Internal Medicine* 141 (2004): 432–40; A. G. Chila, "Pneumonia: Helping Our Bodies Help Themselves," *Consultant* (March 1982): 174–88; C. Feldman, "Pneumonia in the Elderly," *Clinics in Chest Medicine* 20 (1999): 563–73; K. M. Jackson et al., "Effect of Lymphatic and Splenic Pump Tech-

niques on the Antibody Response to Hepatitis B Vaccine: A Pilot Study," *Journal of the American Osteopathic Association* 98 (1998): 155–60; J. A. Knebl et al., "Improving Functional Ability in the Elderly via the Spenser Technique, an Ostepathic Manipulative Treatment: A Randomized, Clinical Trial," *Journal of the American Osteopathic Association* 102 (2002): 347–96; M. Kuchera and A. W. Kuchera, *Osteopathic Considerations in Systemic Dysfunction* (Kirksville, MO: Kirksville College of Osteopathic Medicine Press, 1990), pp. 33–52; R. J. McGovern, ed., *Special Edition on Osteopathy and Aging, Still Review* (Kirksville, MO: A. T. Still University, 2006); D. R. Noll et al., "Effectiveness of a Sham Protocol and Adverse Effects in a Clinical Trial of Osteopathic Manipulative Treatment in Nursing Home Patients," *Journal of the American Osteopathic Association* 104 (2004): 107–13; D. R. Noll et al., "The Effect of Osteopathic Manipulative Treatment on Immune Response to the Influenza Vaccine in Nursing Home Residents: A Pilot Study," *Alternative Therapies in Health and Medicine* 10, no. 4 (2004): 74–76; D. R. Noll and J. C. Johnson, "Revisiting Castlio and Ferris-Swift's Experiments Testing the Effects of Splenic Pump in Normal Individuals," *International Journal of Osteopathic Medicine* 8, no. 4 (2005): 124–30; D. R. Noll et al., "Adjunctive Osteopathic Manipulative Treatment in the Elderly Hospitalized with Pneumonia: A Pilot Study," *Journal of the American Osteopathic Association* 99 (1999): 143–46, 151–52; D. R. Noll et al., "Benefits of Osteopathic Manipulative Treatment for Hospitalized Elderly Patients with Pneumonia," *Journal of the American Osteopathic Association* 100 (2000): 776–82; M. R. Wells et al., "Standard Osteopathic Manipulative Treatment Acutely Improves Gait Performance in Patients with Parkinson's Disease," *Journal of the American Osteopathic Association* 99 (1999): 92–98.

    5. A. T. Still, *Philosophy of Osteopathy* (Indianapolis: American Academy of Osteopathy, 1899); A. T. Still, *The Philosophy and Mechanical Principles of Osteopathy* (Kansas City: Hudson-Kimberly, 1902).

    6. H. H. King, ed., *The Collected Papers of Irvin M. Korr*, vol. 2 (Indianapolis: American Academy of Osteopathy, 1997).

PART 2
THE GUIDING PRINCIPLES

"The more I choose to live in accordance with the laws of nature, the more can I expect to die young when I am very old."

—I. M. Korr

Chapter 2
PRINCIPLE I. INTERACTIVE UNITY
The Oneness of the Person

"The more whole I become, the better my parts operate."

—I. M. Korr

The subtitle of this chapter may seem trite and self-evident, but the implications of that simple phrase—the oneness of the person—are so profound and global in impact, so crucial to health and recovery of health, that we are just beginning to understand the full meaning of the statement that each of us is a unit.

UNITY OF THE BODY

Until recently, only a limited explanation of the unity of the body, although profound in its implications, existed. (I shall shortly explain what I mean by this.) When referring to the unity of the body, one meant that every part was in communication with every other part through the circulating blood and the nervous system. From this perspective, the circulatory and the nervous systems may be regarded as the communication systems that link the numerous tissues and organs together into a single, highly coordinated, self-regulating unit. The nervous system can be compared to high-speed systems, such as the Internet, telephone, radio, and television, while the circulatory system is more comparable to the postal service. The nervous system, via the nerves, conveys electrical impulses, which, in turn, release chemical stimulants and inhibitors known as neurotransmitters, to specific organs and tissues. On the other hand, chemical messengers, such as hormones, are indiscriminately conveyed to all parts of the body by circulating blood and are, in effect, addressed "to whom it may concern." These chemical messengers are manufactured and secreted into the bloodstream by endocrine glands and by certain parts of the brain.

INTERDEPENDENCE IN THE BODY

Every part of the body potentially influences every other part through (1) the nerve impulses it discharges into the central nervous system, which then issues commands to the participating responders, and (2) through the chemical substances it releases into the bloodstream. Every part is affected by the collective messages and signals conveyed by blood and nerves. Linked by the communication systems, all the parts of the body form a community in which each part has a role to play, one that is essential to the welfare of the entire community. Failure of a part to serve adequately for whatever reason affects every other part to some extent. Some are affected more than others, but the body as a whole is affected by the failure. Which part fails and in what way is said to determine the nature of the illness. (As we shall see, there is reason to qualify this conventional wisdom.)

As an example of the interdependence of the different parts of the body, suppose that the function of the heart is impaired in such a way that it does not pump blood in adequate volume. If that were to happen, then the blood flow through the tissues may not be sufficient to deliver required amounts of oxygen and nutrients or to remove the products of metabolism. Tissues would be at once starved and asphyxiated in their own waste products. The brain and kidneys would be given priority over other parts of the body and would, therefore, be protected at the cost of those other parts.

Another example of organ interdependence could be dysfunction of the gastrointestinal tract due to, let us say, an impaired supply of digestive enzymes by the pancreas. Since the role of the digestive system is to reduce the food we eat to simpler substances that can be distributed by the blood and pass into each cell, this dysfunction would also have bodywide consequences. In the cells, these simpler substances, such as glucose, amino acids, and other small molecules, are consumed as fuel for energy or are incorporated into the substance and structure of each cell. Impaired digestion, or faulty absorption of nutrients from the digestive tract, would result in various degrees of undernutrition and malnutrition. Some tissues, such as skeletal muscle and adipose (fatty) tissues, would be sacrificed to nourish others, such as the brain, the heart, and the kidneys.

The kidneys, a third example of interdependence, remove soluble waste products as rapidly as they are produced and brought to the kidneys by the circulating blood. Another role is to control the composition of the blood. If the kidneys do not adequately perform in either of these prescribed roles, renal failure could result, an outcome that would also have bodywide effects.

As a final illustration of interdependence and body unity, consider a situation in which the body produces an abnormally high or low secretion of a hormone, such as insulin, estrogen, or one or more of the hormones of the adrenal cortex. Any unusual change in one hormone would produce effects according to the functions regulated by it and could potentially result in severe bodywide consequences.

Although I have supplied only four examples, these scenarios could be extended to every part of the body. Such an exercise is not necessary for my purpose, but the principle would be the same—namely, every part of the body depends on every other part for the ability to perform its own functions and even for its survival. Most important, and I want to stress this point, the body as a whole also depends on the same principle of interdependence for its proper functioning and survival.

INSEPARABILITY OF BODY AND MIND

In what way, then, is the concept of the unity of the body incomplete? Quite simply, the concept is limited to the body, specifically by the implicit acceptance of the centuries-old concept, usually attributed to philosopher-scientist René Descartes (1596–1650), that the body and the mind are two separate and independent domains.[1]

In view of the accumulated clinical and research evidence of the past three or four decades, this dualistic concept is no longer tenable. The emergence of psychosomatic medicine during the same period reflected the growing recognition in the healing professions that what goes on in the mind (psyche) has powerful influences on what goes on in the body (soma) and that there are psychological effects of physical activities and illnesses. In my opinion, this still reflects dualistic thinking in that it implies interaction between two distinct entities, each doing something to the other. We are, however, increasingly aware that the body and the mind are so inseparable, so pervasive of each other that they can be and must be understood as a single unit. Unfortunately, this kind of thinking is still so new and unfamiliar that we have not yet acquired the appropriate language to express the oneness of body and mind other than through such linguistic devices as body-mind, or bodymind. Regrettably, even these terms preserve the implication of duality. Unfortunately, extending the concept of the unity of the body so that it encompasses a union of the body, mind, and spirit has also been ineffective, especially in view of the lack of clarity, much less consensus, about what is meant by "spirit." Defining what one means by "mind" is difficult enough! It is for these reasons that I prefer the term *unity of the person*, because it conveys the idea of a totally integrated humanity and individuality.

Having said that, it is not my intention to dismiss spirit just because it has been given so many different and often nebulous meanings (as I have personally discovered through decades of extensive reading and countless interviews with people of various religious persuasions). I am aware that many, perhaps most, of my readers have given their own deeply felt meanings to the word or concept of spirit. Therefore, I hope that you will incorporate your own meanings, as you wish, into the concept of the integrated self or person while I focus on bodymind in my discussions.

So how can one speak of the unity of two very different things, where one is as substantial and fleshy as the body and the other is as impalpable, invisible, and private as the mind? As you consider your answer to that question, I will concede that the phenomena that we assign to the realm of the mind, such as consciousness, thought, feelings, beliefs, attitudes, fears, perceptions, hopes, expectations, and so on, have their physiological and behavioral counterparts. I will also concede that bodily and behavioral changes have mental counterparts, such as altered feelings and perceptions. However, it is you, the *person*, who is feeling, perceiving, expecting, and so forth: it is not the mind or the body. Further, it is *I* who feels well or ill, not my mind or body. Therefore, we can state that what goes on in the body and in the mind is conditioned by who the person is and by his or her entire biography.[2]

THE PERSON AS CONTEXT

In short, the person is more—in fact, far more—than the union of the body and the mind (or even of the body, mind, and spirit). This statement is true in the same sense that water is far more than the union of hydrogen and oxygen, as represented by its chemical formula, H_2O, an infinitely simpler example that I will expand on later to illustrate my point. At each higher level of organized complexity, new properties and whole new realms emerge that are not inherent in the parts and their interactions. Once again using the water analogy, nothing that we know about hydrogen or oxygen accounts for the three states of water (liquid, gas, and solid); this includes a consideration of the respective properties, the boiling and freezing points, viscosities, solubilities, and so on, of each state of water. One can say that water incorporates yet transcends oxygen and hydrogen. Therefore, to understand water, we must study water and not merely its components. In the same way, the person incorporates yet transcends the body and the mind.

Similarly, one could make a lifetime career of studying individual cars and drivers but never understand the dynamics of traffic jams. One could study individual bees and still not know how they organize and run their colonies or design and construct their hives. It follows that the understanding of humans incorporates and transcends the study of the mind and the study of the various parts of the body. Echoing this idea, seventeenth-century British poet Alexander Pope wrote in "An Essay on Man" that "the proper study of Mankind is Man."[3] In the context of this discussion, I would propose that the proper study of human health and illness is the study of the whole person.

Relative to health and illness, this brings us to what is perhaps the most important implication of the unity of the person. The person is the context, the environment in which all the parts of the body, including the brain, live and function. Everything about the person, such as his or her entire history, nutrition, upbringing, attitudes, talents, behavior, beliefs, use (or abuse) of the body and mind, quality of interpersonal relationships, physical and sociocultural environments, and so on and so forth, enters into determining the quality of the operation of the different parts of the body.

REDUCTIONISM AND BIOMEDICAL RESEARCH

This concept stands in sharp contrast to the prevailing perspective in biomedical research and in healthcare usually characterized by the terms *mechanistic* and *reductionist*. The underlying premise in the reductionist strategy or paradigm is that the whole organism, the human in this case, can be explained only in terms of its component parts.

From this viewpoint, therefore, the best way and perhaps the only way to understand humans and their frailties is to take them apart and reduce them to their components. Each component is then minutely studied in the laboratory. Only then, according to this view, can we understand the human, how the human goes wrong, how to set him right again, and what to do to the faulty part to cure the disease and restore the person to health.[4]

This strategy has, of course, been enormously productive, providing knowledge about biological mechanisms that later became the basis for many of our greatest medical advances. I would venture to say that this strategy is at the heart of so-called scientific medicine. (Regrettably, what often passes for scientific medicine is the unscientific use of the products of science.) There is no denying that the reductionist study of the human has an important role in continued medical progress or that the quality of the parts' functions profoundly influences the health and clinical course of the individual. This, however, is only part of the picture. To revisit a previous example, it is analogous, in an infinitely more complex way, to studying hydrogen and oxygen under the assumption that one is learning about water.

It is important to remember that most of our knowledge about component parts, processes, and mechanisms has been the product of research on lower animals. What is missing in the reductionist paradigm, as it seeks to apply that knowledge to human biology as well as human health and disease, is the human context in which the components function. Included are not only the innumerable varying features and modifying circumstances unique to the human species and human life, but also those unique to the individual human.

The life circumstances in and around each person as well as the unique manner in which they respond and adapt to those circumstances has a powerful, and often critical, health-related influence on how well the component parts, processes, and mechanisms serve the individual. Reinserting the component parts into the whole-person context completes the reductionistic paradigm.

In this chapter, I have tried to establish the unity of the body and mind as well as their incorporation in the person. Nevertheless, because the body and the mind require different technologies and languages for exploration and explication, I will separate them temporarily in succeeding chapters and reunite them again later.

NOTES

1. A. R. Demasio, *Descartes' Error: Emotion, Reason, and the Human Brain* (New York: Putnam, 1994).

2. J. LeDoux, *Synaptic Self: How Our Brains Become Who We Are* (Middlesex: Penguin, 2002).

3. A. Pope, "An Essay on Man," in *Alexander Pope Selected Works*, ed. L. Kronenberger (New York: Modern Library, 1951), pp. 97–137.

4. M. Ben-Ari, *Just a Theory: Exploring the Nature of Science* (Amherst, NY: Prometheus Books, 2005); D. Deutsch, *The Fabric of Reality* (New York: Penguin, 1998).

Chapter 3

PRINCIPLE II.
STRUCTURE-FUNCTION

The Primary Machinery

"Intellect, education, training, and even the noblest ethical, moral, and religious principles have value only insofar as they are expressed in our behavior."

—I. M. Korr

THE DOING OF WHAT HUMANS DO: LIFE IS MOTION

Of all the parts of the body, which is the most important? This question is as silly as asking who is the most important person in the community. Is it the schoolteachers, the police, the trash collectors, the city council? Obviously, all the parts are important for the healthy life of the community. Equally obvious, some organs, like the heart, are indispensable for survival, while others, like the spleen, a leg, the cerebral cortex, or the reproductive organs are not. While not necessary for survival, their loss, however, would diminish the quality of life.

Throughout its history, medicine has attached the greatest importance to the internal organs. In recent decades, many remarkable instruments and techniques have been developed for the functional evaluation and treatment of the internal organs. Accordingly, we now have subspecialties of internal medicine, such as cardiology, gastroenterology, and nephrology. This emphasis on the viscera has of course yielded some of our greatest medical advances, but these great strides forward have been at the cost of the main bulk of the body. In particular, the study of the musculoskeletal system, which comprises muscles, bones, joints, ligaments, tendons, and other connective tissues, has suffered the most. Instead, the musculoskeletal system has been set aside as the province of specialists in orthopedics, physical and rehabilitative medicine, and sports medicine. As one physician put it, "Sometimes we seem to think of the musculoskeletal system as a vehicle for carting our insides to the internist."

Another consequence of the medical preoccupation with our internal organs is that life comes to be seen as a composite of visceral functions. That is a fallacy. Human life, a person's activity and behavior, does not consist of such components as peristalsis, cardiac output, or kidney function. These are simply examples of what organs do.

Human life is expressed as human beings doing things that humans do. Generally, whatever humans do, they do with muscles, and most of those muscles are pulling on bony levers. Every human action consists of coordinated contractions and relaxations of numerous muscles. Human behavior is ultimately the complex, continually changing, orchestrated patterns of muscular contractions and relaxations. In short, the ultimate instrument of human action and behavior is the musculoskeletal system. It is the means through which we express our humanity and our individuality.

Further, the musculoskeletal system is the means by which we manifest in our own way every human quality, be it intellect, curiosity, creativity, compassion, imagination, humor, or love. Every feeling, fear, hope, or aspiration has its ultimate expression through muscular action even if only by communication to others through language, gesture, or grimace. Intellect, education, training, and even the noblest ethical, moral, and religious principles have value only insofar as they are expressed in our behavior as the things we do for, with, and to each other, to other creatures, and to the planet we share. Behavior is possible only through the instrumentality of the musculoskeletal system. Every act, utterance, written word, deed, posture, caress, glance, gesture, artistic creation, musical performance, or facial expression (whether it be a frown, smile, smirk, or quizzical raising of an eyebrow) is the product of muscular contraction and relaxation. Even breathing, eating, elimination, sex, and reproduction require the motor power of the musculoskeletal system. Life is, indeed, motion.

THE COMMAND CENTER

All the things that humans do are, of course, organized by the central nervous system through the patterns of signals (impulses) conveyed to the muscles by the motor nerve fibers, the great majority of which originate in the spinal cord. The motor nerves fire their impulses to the muscles in response to impulses reaching them from the brain and from numerous sensory receptors throughout the body. Most body receptors are strategically placed in muscles, joints, tendons, ligaments, and skin. In fact, most commands issued by the spinal cord, including its blood vessels, are directed to the musculoskeletal system, and most sensory input to the spinal cord is from the musculoskeletal system. Clearly, control of motion and posture, that is, muscular action, is a major part of the business of the nervous system. For all the above reasons, I have come to agree with A. T. Still, the founder of osteopathy, who viewed the musculoskeletal system as the "primary machinery of human life."[1]

THE MAIN CONSUMERS

As the motors of the musculoskeletal system, the muscles of the body may be viewed as the body's main consumers. I say this about the muscles not only because of their mass, which is a major part of body weight, but also because of their high-energy demands for the services enumerated in the preceding paragraph. Moreover, their requirements vary widely from moment to moment according to what the person is doing and in what environment. In short, the total economy of the body must be continually tuned to the high and variable requirements of the musculoskeletal system (and of the environment). Much of the tuning is done by the autonomic (vegetative) nervous system. It is evident that in its varying activities, the musculoskeletal system continually challenges and disturbs the dynamic balance and relative constancy of the internal environment in which all the cells of the body carry out their respective activities.

THE MAINTENANCE AND SERVICE DEPARTMENT

What, then, is the function of the internal organs with which physicians are so preoccupied? From the viewpoint expressed above, their collective role is that of maintenance and service—the "boiler works" as one of my students described it—for the primary machinery. Circulation, respiration, metabolism, and so on are responsible for meeting the logistical requirements of the musculoskeletal system by (1) supplying the fuels and nutrients required for energy, growth, and self-maintenance; (2) carting off and disposing of the products of metabolism; (3) dissipating the heat that is generated and regulating the body temperature; (4) controlling the environments in which the cells live; (5) defending and protecting against harmful substances and organisms; and (6) contributing to self-repair. Of course, in providing these services to the musculoskeletal system, the internal organs are at the same time providing the same services for each other and for the body as a whole, including the entire nervous system.

THE NATURE OF ILLNESS

The preceding perspective provides a better understanding of the essential nature of illness. Illness results from, and indeed is, the disparity between the requirements of the primary machinery and the degree to which those requirements are met by the maintenance and service department.[2] When the demands of the musculoskeletal system significantly and for too long exceed the capacity of the services, then muscular effort, even supporting one's weight, becomes difficult if not impossible, and we take to bed. In other words, therapeutic rest is automatically enforced. The disparity between the two systems may be due to (1) sustained, intense emotional and behavioral demand (including diffuse muscular tension); (2) structural, postural, and functional disturbances in the musculoskeletal system; (3) inadequacy or aberration of some visceral, metabolic, or other internal function; or (4) faulty communication between the musculoskeletal system and other systems.

In the preceding chapter, I stressed that all parts of the body are in continual communication with each other. Obviously, the musculoskeletal system is a major participant in this interchange. Hence, disturbances in musculoskeletal function may have adverse effects on other organs; conversely, aberrations in visceral, endocrine, metabolic, or other internal functions will be reflected in the musculoskeletal system. This has important implications for human health because the human framework is uniquely vulnerable to gravitational forces, as will be explained in chapter 8.[3]

THE PRICE OF INACTIVITY

The concept of musculoskeletal primacy has other important implications for health, especially for older persons. When physical inactivity becomes habitual, as it too often does in the older population, then the challenge and the variety of challenges demanded of the cardiovascular, respiratory, renal, and other systems are greatly reduced. The internal organs, called on only for basic maintenance, undergo progressive diminution both of their functional capacities and of their reserve capacity to meet sudden or prolonged demand.

The familiar saying "Use it or lose it" is especially meaningful in this capacity. The change is not unlike the atrophy from disuse and the withering that is seen in the inactive musculoskeletal system in the muscles, bones, and connective tissues. A vicious circle ensues: The longer the inactivity, the greater the loss of functional capacity; the greater that loss, the more difficult it becomes to move, thus the greater the inactivity. This cycle continues until movement, even body support, becomes impossible. The person is then said to be in heart failure, respiratory failure, kidney failure, or some other type of disease. Conversely, remaining active throughout life sustains and even enhances the capacity for activity, the potential of the person, and his or her enjoyment of life.

A comprehensive review of the consequences of inactivity for persons both young and old can be found in the book *Inactivity: Physiological Effects*.[4] Experimental studies, some of which I personally observed in the course of my research during World War II, have shown that the deleterious effects of inactivity, such as prolonged bed rest, on young people are very similar to those seen in the older population. The young people even began to *look* old!

SUMMARY

I have singled out the musculoskeletal system for this long discussion not because it is more important than the other systems (an absurd concept as we have seen), but in order to counterbalance the prevailing emphasis in medical thought and practice on the other systems. My purpose has also been to explain its place in the total economy of the body and its role as the instrument by which we express ourselves. As that instrument of expression, it is inert and valueless apart from the mind that puts it to use. In the same way, the mind has no means of overt expression apart from the musculoskeletal system.

NOTES

1. A. T. Still, *Osteopathy, Research and Practice* (1910; repr., Seattle: Eastland Press, 1992), pp. 22–23; A. T. Still, *Philosophy of Osteopathy* (Indianapolis: American Academy of Osteopathy, 1899).

2. R. M. Nesse and G. C. Williams, *Why We Get Sick: The New Science of Darwinian Medicine* (New York: Vintage, 1994).

3. J. C. Eccles, *Evolution of the Brain: Creation of the Self* (New York: Routledge, 1989).

4. H. Sandler, *Inactivity: Physiological Effects*, ed. J. Vernikos (New York: Academic Press, 1986).

Chapter 4

PRINCIPLE III.
VIS MEDICATRIX NATURAE

The Only True Healthcare System

"To find health should be the object of the doctor. Anyone can find disease."

—A. T. Still

GETTING WELL VERSUS MAKING WELL

The ancient Latin phrase *vis medicatrix naturae* reflects man's early awareness of nature's healing power, something with which each of us is endowed. This healing power manifests itself, as it did to Hippocrates and others thousands of years ago, in many ways. For example, when you accidentally cut your finger, alarmed though you may be at that moment by the pain and dripping blood, you nevertheless count on the certainty that you will not bleed to death. You expect that the bleeding will stop, thanks to your body's built-in clotting mechanism. Moreover, in most circumstances, you have no fear that infection will occur or that the damaged tissues will not heal. You may choose, however, to treat the injury with an antiseptic and a bandage for double assurance.

Consider, too, that even broken bones heal without intervention, although keeping the fragments aligned and immobilized by a cast, splint, or other means may be necessary. It is also true that one can recover from much more serious wounds and injuries, such as those that occur in warfare, traffic accidents, and violent crimes. Whatever the medical or surgical assistance required, ultimate healing is that performed by the enormously complex biological mechanisms subsumed under *vis medicatrix naturae*.[1]

Similarly, when we have caught a cold or a bad case of the flu, miserable as we may feel, there is usually no doubt in our minds that the illness is self-limiting and will run its course. We are certain that we will recover because our inherent immune and other defensive and restorative mechanisms are always at work. Even in these and other infectious diseases when medication is administered that slows or arrests proliferation of the pathogenic bacteria or viruses, it is the patient's body mechanisms that destroy and eliminate the infection, and it is the body that repairs the damage done by the infection.[2]

The same is essentially true of other, more serious diseases, including cancers, where spontaneous recovery is known to take place.[3] As necessary and helpful as medication, surgery, radiation, or other medical intervention may have been, the recovery is ultimately the patient's own achievement. It is not the physician or the treatment that makes the patient well; it is the patient who gets well.

Healing, recovery, and cure come from within. The physician and the physician's technology can facilitate and disencumber these processes by removing impediments to their effectiveness, but the physician cannot do the healing for the patient. I do not mean in any way to diminish the role of the physician or the treatment; both are often essential and even crucial to the patient's improvement. My purpose is to place their roles in proper perspective.

DEFENSE AGAINST EXTERNAL THREATS

What about all the colds, flus, and other illnesses that we do not get? Are our healing mechanisms idle and dormant during those long periods, waiting, like firemen, for the alarm to sound? Or are they continually walking the beat as policemen (used to) do? After all, we are surrounded by pathogenic organisms. We are even host to many of them, which live in the upper respiratory tract and elsewhere. Fortunately, it is only occasionally, rarely, or never that they are permitted by our defense mechanisms to proliferate and make us ill. So maybe the next time you catch a cold, instead of asking yourself if the person who sneezed in your direction on the elevator is responsible for making you ill, you should instead ask if you got sick because your guard was down for some reason.

It was my privilege over a period of many years as a professor of medical physiology to make an annual observation that is relevant to this question. One hundred new students came each fall to northeast Missouri to begin their medical studies. They came from all parts of the United States and from other countries. After my first few years, I learned to expect with each first-year class that, beginning in late November, coughing, sneezing, and nose blowing would become more and more intrusive in the classroom, and that absenteeism would suddenly increase and continue almost until the holiday recess.

Further, it was my consistent observation that the victims were in the minority. The conventional medical questions that would have been asked concerning this observation were, "What went wrong with those students?" and "What was the infectious agent responsible for the epidemic?" I learned that much more fruitful questions to ask are "What was right with the others?" "What advantage, what resources did they have that the victims lacked that kept the healthy students well even though they shared the same climate, the same work environment, and even the same germs with the coughers and sneezers for long hours each day?" and "Why were their protective mechanisms more effective?" A final and quite pertinent question I would include is "What can be learned from the healthy students that could be shared with the others?"

In addition to our natural defensive mechanisms that protect us from colds and flus, other bodily mechanisms protect us against poisonous and harmful chemicals we ingest with our food and drink or absorb through our skin and lungs. This mechanism works in several ways. For instance, the immune system disarms foreign proteins, while the liver, kidneys, and intestinal tract convert those proteins into harmless substances and eliminate them from the body.

GUARDING THE INTERNAL ENVIRONMENT

This leads me to a new series of questions I would like you to consider. Are these protective, healing, and recuperative mechanisms effective only against threats, invasions, and insults from without? What about those threats originating within—endogenously? As a physiologist, I have some knowledge and much awe of the enormous complexity, the reliability, and the precision of the body's many regulatory mechanisms. It is through those mechanisms that humans can live in and adapt to environmental extremes (temperature, humidity, barometric pressure) and sustain themselves with food and drink of diverse chemical composition and degrees of acidity or alkalinity (pH). As a researcher studying war-related biomedical problems during World War II, I was personally exposed in experimental chambers each day to one or more of the following simulated conditions of (1) extremely high altitudes, (2) the Arctic, (3) the jungle, (4) or desert climates, without any apparent ill effects. However, the cells of our body can function and survive only in an internal environment that is maintained within or quickly returned to very narrow limits of temperature, chemical composition, osmotic pressure, and pH. This readjustment must be accomplished no matter what the variations in external environment or the activities of the person.

The internal environment of the cells consists of thin fluid layers that bathe the cells. This interstitial fluid is essentially a filtrate of blood plasma, with the filtration taking place across the capillary walls. Maintenance of the constancy of the internal environment, whatever the external environment or activity of the person, is called homeostasis, a term coined early in the twentieth century by Harvard physiologist Walter B. Cannon.[4] This relative constancy, or steady state, is the product of dynamic equilibrium. For example, the concentration of glucose or oxygen in the blood remains within narrow limits because it is continually replenished as rapidly as it is consumed by the cells. Carbon dioxide is removed as rapidly as it is produced by the cells, and red blood cells, which continually wear out in great numbers, are replaced at the same rate by fresh cells. Body temperature remains constant because heat is dissipated to the external environment as rapidly as it is generated by cell metabolism and physical activity. In cold weather, the heat generated by shivering is also lost to the environment.

In view of the truly dynamic quality of these thousands of bodily equilibria, I regret that Cannon did not choose the term *homeokinesis* rather than homeostasis. The mental image I have for these processes is that of a rapidly flowing mountain stream whose level at each point is constant because outflow is balanced by inflow from the source. Constancy, or fixity, of levels is due to a dynamic balance between opposite fluxes. For this reason, I taught my students to think of homeostasis as a manifestation of the *law of fixity—fluxity*.

THE ROUTINE MIRACLES

Let me explain through example the reason for my awe as I study these self-regulatory, homeostatic mechanisms. In the regulation of arterial blood pressure, blood sugar, oxygen, pH, body temperature, and so on, there are hundreds of component mechanisms, countless variables and impinging factors, and numerous sensing, signaling, and feedback components. In a system with such immense complexity, the opportunities for malfunction and breakdown are so enormous and, seemingly, so highly probable (witness NASA's recurrent problems) that it never ceases to amaze me, not that dysfunction does occur, but that it occurs so seldom. It is, indeed, a wonder to me that everybody doesn't have hyper- or hypotension, hypoxia, hyper- or hypoglycemia, hyper- or hypothermia, acidosis, or alkalosis!

In the same way, when I contemplate the billions upon billions of cell divisions that occur as a fertilized ovum eventually becomes an adult human being and the corresponding numbers of opportunities for chromosomal, genetic, and developmental abnormalities, I cannot help but be amazed that everybody doesn't have cancer or isn't a grotesque monstrosity. These are but a few of the countless miracles routinely performed each day by *vis medicatrix naturae*. It is not only the body's own healing system; it is a real health maintenance organization. It is truly a complete and preventive healthcare system.

THE CAUSES OF HEALTH

Understandably, the profession of medicine is so preoccupied with what is wrong and with seeking the causes and cures of this or that disease that we overlook the infinitely greater promise in finding the causes of what is right; the causes of nonhypertension, nondiabetes, nonulcer, nonflu, non–heart disease. In short, we overlook finding the cause of nondisease. In the same way and transcending nondisease, we overlook finding the causes of health. What is really required of us is that we look upon health itself as a remarkable phenomenon and one in much need of research.

This book is not the place to examine in detail the various protective, immunological, detoxifying, healing, recuperative, restorative, regenerative, compensatory, and regulatory homeostatic mechanisms. It is also not the place to do more than identify the comprehensive protective role of the brain as director and coordinator of these mechanisms as well as of our behavior. For my purposes, it is enough to say at this point that when these mechanisms are permitted and enabled to function optimally and without impediment, their inevitable product is what we call health. Their natural tendency is always toward health and the recovery of health. Further, these mechanisms are the very source of health. Each person, as we shall see, has considerable influence on the quality of their function and, therefore, on her or his health.

THE PHYSICIAN WITHIN AND THE BODY'S OWN PHARMACY

My favorite metaphor for this marvelous assemblage of mechanisms is the "physician within." As has been discovered in recent decades, the internal physician has available a large and diverse pharmacy of the body's own medicines, dubbed *endocoids* by my former colleague Harbans Lal, PhD.[5] Scores of these endocoids are manufactured in various parts of the brain. Because of their origin and chemical nature, they are known as *neuropeptides*. Some of the best-known neuropeptides that the general public would be aware of are the endorphins, chemical cousins of morphine. It is interesting to note that neuropeptides have diverse influences on the body besides pain perception. For example, they influence the immune system, sexual behavior, food intake, mood, and other aspects of cerebral activity. (Some of the same peptides are manufactured elsewhere in the body, such as in the digestive tract. Indeed, they seem to have originated there and to have been adopted later by the evolving brain.)

The manufacture and release of neuropeptides are influenced by a person's psychic makeup and behavior, and vice versa. They are generally regarded as part of the cement that binds body and mind into a single entity. It is through the discovery of this neurochemical two-way communication between brain and immune system that the new field of biomedical research known as psychoneuroimmunology (PNI) has evolved.

There are many different types of the body's own medicines besides neuropeptides; some of them originate in various organs and glands as well as in the immune system. These other bodily medicines include interferon, a sort of versatile antibiotic; digoxin-like substances that influence cardiac activity; immune substances known as the interleukins; renin, an enzyme produced by the kidney that is important in the regulation of arterial blood pressure; the prostaglandins, which have assorted regulatory and corrective actions; and hormones that influence inflammatory processes, electrolyte balance, and water excretion.

The physician within, in effect, makes its own diagnoses, writes its own prescriptions, manufactures its own medicines, and administers each dose. Further, it completes this process without the undesirable side effects that are so common with externally administered medication. The physician within is the only true healthcare system upon which all others depend, and without it, the others are impotent. It is unfortunate that the numerous components of this enormously complex and competent system, such as the control of circulation, respiration, immunity, acid-base balance, temperature, and so on, are so scattered among the scientific disciplines that its total grandeur, its human context, and its relevance to human health are obscured.

The next chapter looks briefly into the care and nurturing of the physician within and into the relationship between the quality of that care, on the one hand, and health and illness, on the other.

NOTES

1. R. Ader, D. L. Felten, and N. Cohen, eds., *Psychoneuroimmunology*, 3rd ed., 2 vols. (San Diego: Academic Press, 2001); J. Borysenko, *Minding the Body, Mending the Mind* (Reading, MA: Addison-Wesley, 1987); S. Freier, ed., *The Neuroendocrine—Immune Network* (Boca Raton, FL: CRC Press, 1989); S. S. Hall, "A Molecular Code Links Emotions, Mind, and Health," *Smithsonian* 20 (1989): 62–71; J. K. Kiecolt-Glaser et al., "Psychoneuroimmunology and Psychosomatic Medicine: Back to the Future," *Psychosomatic Medicine* 64 (2002): 15–28; I. M. Korr, "History of Medicine and the Concept of Endocoids," in *Endocoids*, ed. H. Lal, F. LaBella, and J.

Lane (New York: Alan R. Liss, 1985); C. B. Pert, "The Wisdom of the Receptors," *Advances* 3 (1986): 8–16; C. B. Pert, *The Molecules of Emotion: The Science behind Mind-Body Medicine* (New York: Scribner, 1997); R. Ader, N. Cohen, and D. L. Felten, eds., *Brain, Behavior and Immunity*, vol. 3 (New York: Academic Press, 1989).

2. S. Locke and D. Colligan, *The Healer Within: The New Medicine of Mind & Body* (New York: Mentor, 1986).

3. C. Hirshberg and M. I. Barasch, *Remarkable Recovery: What Extraordinary Healings Tell Us about Getting Well and Staying Well* (New York: Riverhead, 1995); A. Weil, *Spontaneous Healing* (New York: Ballantine, 1995).

4. W. B. Cannon, *Wisdom of the Body* (Gloucester, MA: Peter Smith, 1963).

5. I. M. Korr, "History of Medicine and the Concept of Endocoids," *Progress in Clinical and Biological Research* 192 (1985): 1–4; H. Lal, F. LaBella, and J. Lane, eds., *Endocoids* (New York: Wiley-Liss, 1985).

Chapter 5

PRINCIPLE IV.
MEANING DRIVES EXPECTANCY

Take Care of the Physician Within and the Physician Within Will Take Care of You

"Upon completing the grieving that follows each gate-closing or loss in my life, I begin to prepare for the new openings and gains that follow."

—I. M. Korr

In order to stress their message, the paragraphs that follow are set in a chapter of their own rather than being tacked on to the preceding chapter. It is my intention that this chapter convey the strategy or motivation for implementing the foregoing three closely linked principles. Specifically, I want to clearly delineate the meaning and expectancy of the unity of the person, the structure-function of the musculoskeletal system, and the body's inherent protective, regulatory, and restorative mechanisms. I see the principles I describe in this section as the basis for genuine whole-person healthcare. I also see them as distinguished from and complementing organ-focused disease care.

As was outlined in my discussion of the first principle in chapter 2, the person is the environment and the context in which all the body parts live, function, and serve that person. This includes all the cells and all the tissues and organs that they form. Lest we forget, the structure and function of the musculoskeletal system (principle II) and all the interactive components that compose the healing power of nature (principle III) are also an integral part of this discussion of principle IV.

How well all these parts operate and serve the person is determined by the quality of the environment provided by the person. That is, how well the parts function is determined by the life that the person *chooses* and is enabled to live. Virtually every factor and circumstance in that life either enhances or diminishes the quality of life, including one's expectations and goals regarding health. Some factors are the individual's genetic endowment; the individual's entire history, beginning with the conditions of his or her conception, fetal development, and birth; the individual's beliefs, attitudes, values, and priorities absorbed from family and culture; the individual's behavior, nutrition, use of bodymind, and abuse of bodymind; and the opportunities and total milieu provided by the society in which the individual lives.

From this perspective, I would like to propose the following four levels inherent in total healthcare:

- The first is the biological level. This includes the cells, tissues, organs, and organ systems; the nervous system and brain; and the musculoskeletal system. Principles I through III have application with this level.

- The second is the individual/personal level. The most direct and ultimate responsibility for maintaining, enhancing, and even recovering health is centered here. This level postulates that one must be motivated, educated, and enabled to take meaningful responsibility for one's health. Principle IV applies to this level.

- The third is the community level. This includes significant others, one's family, and the community at large. I would like to point out that it is the community's responsibility to support and allow health-enhancing behaviors among its citizens. This level also includes the physician and the healthcare system. It is their job to teach the art and science of healthful living. In treating the ill, they should use available knowledge and technology that will utilize, support, and enhance a patient's own capacity for recovery. Further, they should strive to remove the impediments interfering with the individual's bodily functioning and, above all, to do no harm to that individual's bodily capacity.

- The fourth and final level is the cultural and subcultural. This incorporates values regarding society's responsibility to (1) provide whatever is required to educate, motivate, and enable the individual to take personal responsibility; (2) guard the quality of the natural environment; (3) create the socioeconomic conditions with which and in which each individual is guaranteed life, liberty, and the pursuit of health and happiness; and (4) enable, motivate, and teach children and youths to adopt healthful ways of living as an essential social responsibility.

Of the above four levels of total healthcare, only the first and second are discussed in detail in this book. The other two levels are beyond the scope of my discussion; however, resources are available for learning more about the third and fourth levels.[1] I do hasten to emphasize that each of us has the obligation, and certainly the opportunity, to do whatever we can to persuade and motivate those who share the other two sets of responsibilities to perform their duties to the fullest on behalf of personal and public health. The means for fulfilling these responsibilities might include direct requests to healthcare providers. They could include exerting our influence on governmental policy, legislation, and implementation by a citizen's use of voice and vote; by communication with elected representatives and agencies in local, state, and federal government; and by joining and supporting organizations dedicated to guarding the environment and to improving public health as well as the general human condition.

To summarize, these four principles, with roots in ancient history, have been likened elsewhere to Aristotle's explanation of the various ways to understand reality.[2] While only the body and the mind are directly addressed in this book, the principles apply to the whole person—mind, body, and spirit. Principle I, interactive unity or the oneness of the person, describes how the various parts of a person's mind, body, or spirit are interactive, so health or disease in one part can affect other parts. Principle II, structure-function interdependency, which is best exemplified by the primary machinery of the musculoskeletal system, shows what is needed and that restoring natural structures helps function. In turn, various types of functioning can affect structures of the mind, body, and spirit. This includes health habits and ways of thinking and feeling. Principle III discusses nature's pharmacy and how a person's mind, body, and spirit have natural predispositions toward self-adjusting or adapting to restore health. Finally, and most important for this chapter, the fourth principle of meaning driving expectancy involves the final cause or intention of the individual to *seek* or *allow* health. Taking care of the physician within so that the physician within will take care of you involves seeing health with understanding and meaning in order to transcend some aspects of human nature. In part 4 of this book, I will discuss *changing the mind* and paths to *commitment, discipline,* and *motivation* that I came to understand through my personal transformation. In the meantime, our next step is to understand those factors peculiar to the human species and human life that render us uniquely vulnerable to illness and infirmity, and even to extinction.

NOTES

1. F. Borrell-Carrio, A. L. Suchman, and R. M. Epstein, "The Biopsychosocial Model 25 Years Later: Principles, Practice, and Scientific Inquiry," *Annals of Family Medicine* 2 (2004): 576–82; G. Engel, "The Need for a New Medical Model: A Challenge for Biomedicine," *Science* 196 (1977): 129–36; G. Engel, "The Clinical Application of the Biopsychosocial Model," *American Journal of Psychiatry* 137 (1980): 534–44; R. M. Frankel, T. E. Quill, and S. H. McDaniel, eds., *The Biopsychosocial Approach: Past, Pre-*

sent, and Future (Rochester, NY: University of Rochester Press, 2003); J. R. Millenson, *Mind Matters* (Seattle: Eastland Press, 1995).

2. J. J. McGovern and R. J. McGovern, *Your Healer Within: A Unified Field Theory of Healthcare* (Tucson, AZ: Fenestra, 2003).

PART 3

ORIGINS OF
HUMAN VULNERABILITY

"To get out of the woods, I first go into the woods."
—I. M. Korr

Chapter 6

INDIVIDUAL PATHS TO HEALTH AND ILLNESS

"That which is spurned as chaff by others is often grist for my mill."

—I. M. Korr

HEALTH AND HUMAN DIVERSITY

As the frequently heard term *human nature* implies, all humans have much in common both biologically and behaviorally. Yet every individual alive today, long dead, or yet to be born plays, has played, or will play absolutely unique variations on these basic, human themes. Although human diversity is universally recognized, that recognition has had little influence on the everyday care of the sick or on the prevention of illness. The terms *idiosyncratic* and *idiopathic*, often offered as explanations of a patient's peculiar symptoms or reactions to medication, are merely fancy terms to conceal our ignorance.[1]

The advances in recent decades of biomedical knowledge about some of today's common and deadly diseases as well as their successful treatment have been encouraging. Risk factors statistically shown to be more or less causally related to some of the diseases have been identi-

73

fied, such as smoking to lung cancer and fat consumption to coronary artery disease. Personal control of some of these risk factors has had a significant impact on the incidence and severity of these diseases.[2]

Despite this burgeoning knowledge and technology, however, we still have little understanding of how individual differences relate to differences in susceptibility to illness and, even less, to levels of health. After all, it is not only the differences in our genetic programming but also virtually every aspect of and influence on our individual lives that determines the physiological paths that we follow.

In short, human biography and human biology are inseparably related. Biographical features determine our attained levels of health, general vulnerability, susceptibility to particular ailments, quality of our lives, and the time and manner of our dying. Each of us knows people who live long, active, almost illness-free lives. At the other extreme, we also know people who live short lives filled with illness, pain, and disability. There is much to be learned from the study of the superbly healthy. For instance, we need to ask and answer the question: What is it about the superbly healthy and the circumstances of their lives that may account for their good fortune? We are too much inclined to shrug off the good fortune as the luck of the draw in the cosmic gene pool, but we have reached a point in human existence when this answer can no longer suffice.

THE CAUSES OF HEALTH

Unfortunately and understandably, we are so preoccupied with sickness and the study of disease that we neglect the study of high-level health as a phenomenon in and of itself. To counter this disproportionate balance, we need to move our attention more and more to the other end of the health spectrum; we need to be concerned with the causes of health as much as we are with the causes of disease.[3]

There is much to be learned from the study of those who (like myself until my forties) are not yet sick with known diseases but who are also not well. Indeed, this group constitutes the vast reservoir in which the chronic degenerative diseases so rampant today are spawned. It is increasingly recognized that these chronic diseases, especially prevalent among the aged but also common in the young, are largely products of what is usually referred to as lifestyle, something that is always subject to ameliorative change. Hence, the importance of identifying the health-enhancing secrets of healthy people and of studying preclinical, lower levels of health (found in such conditions as chronic fatigue, backache, headache, stiffness, anxiety, depression, digestive problems, and just "not feeling good") for their predictive value and amenability to protective correction.[4]

Numerous studies of medical histories have yielded important insights into various populations or cohorts. Examples of some of those cohorts are workers in an industrial plant, executives in a corporation, or people in a given community, institution, or ethnic group.[5] In longitudinal studies of these groups, over time a majority of the incidents of illness are found to have been concentrated in a minority of the people, while at the other extreme another minority has been virtually free of illness.[6] Furthermore, the patterns of illness in the less fortunate minority are remarkably constant for each individual, except that over time the illnesses tend to become more and more serious and involve more and more parts of the body. Also reflected in most of these studies is the fact that while medical care may have had palliative (symptom-relieving) or remedial effects on individual incidents of illness, it has had little or no effect on the patterns of illness. That is, it has had little effect on general vulnerability.[7]

Challenging questions about such issues began to excite me early in my career as a teacher at an osteopathic medical school. An early stimulus was the observation mentioned in chapter 4 that only a third or a fourth of the students in each first-year class succumbed to upper respiratory infections as winter approached. Instead of speculating, as was and is customary, about the infectious microbes causing the illness and how they may have been caught by the victims in the first place, various questions about the healthy students came to my mind and are reiterated here for emphasis: (1) What enabled the nonvictims to escape infection despite their exposure to the same infectious agents? (2) What protective advantage did they have over the others? (3) In what way(s) was their physiology superior? (4) What could be learned from them that might benefit their less fortunate classmates?

The usual glib answers, such as "They have a higher resistance to disease" or "They have more competent immune systems," only begged the question. Wherein was the higher resistance? What *made* the immune system more competent, and what kept it that way?

I found these questions disquieting because the subject of physiology, as usually taught in medical schools, offers little insight into these issues despite the fact that they are so crucial to human health. Even though physiology purports to be human physiology, its subject matter has largely (and with good reason!) been gathered and supported by research on "lower" animals. We humans do share countless features with other mammals at the molecular, cellular, tissue, and even organ levels, and we have learned an enormous amount about what goes on in the human body from animal research. But this is not to say that the human context is therefore irrelevant. In view of our diversity, even the differences among us are not irrelevant.

Having been taught and then having taught about *the* heart, *the* stomach, *the* kidneys, and so forth, I suddenly became aware that these were abstractions, mere conceptual models, which do not exist in isolation in nature. These models of hearts, stomachs, kidneys, and so forth, all observe universal laws that exist only in the minds of teachers and their students. Each heart is different in some ways from all other hearts (each stomach from all other stomachs, and so on) according to the person it serves and in whose body it functions and has functioned. Only when we begin to understand these individual differences or contexts for function can we begin to understand why some hearts (or other organs and processes) become impaired in different ways in early or midlife, while others go on serving the person well for eighty to one hundred years or more.

The latter group shows us quite clearly that good and even excellent function of the body's organs at an advanced age is within the human potential. Indeed, a former director of the National Institute on Aging (one of the National Institutes of Health), in a 1996 review article, stated that research is leading to the conclusion that in most organ systems in humans there is the biological potential for older individuals to maintain the same function as young adults into their later years.[8] Further, the author points out that the human brain is among the most durable of the organs. (I will talk more about the brain later.)

FUTURE CASE HISTORIES

Returning to my previous puzzlement about the "constitutional" differences (another term that conceals our ignorance) between the two segments of each freshman osteopathic medical class, I wondered how their state of sickness or health might relate to differences in their future health-and-disease patterns as well as their longevity. I began to speculate about the future clinical histories of friends and colleagues whom I knew well and with whose personal lives I was familiar. I remember preparing and delivering a lecture that I titled "Three Future Case Histories" to a meeting of internal medicine specialists. Two of the three persons I had chosen as my subjects for this exercise in prognostication were my closest collaborators and fellow physician-scientists who joined the department soon after I assumed the chairmanship. The third person in that case history was myself, more than ten years their senior.

Because of my family history, I had predicted that I would be the first to die, after one or more heart attacks. I predicted that my two colleagues would survive me by many years, one because of his seemingly tranquil, conservative, and contemplative lifestyle, and the other because of his high energy, self-confidence, and athletic ability.

I was totally wrong. Both of my colleagues died in their early fifties, whereas I continued to enjoy life into my nineties. How could I have been so wrong? Easily. My forecasts were made before I had come to appreciate the implications to my own health of the guidelines set forth in the earlier chapters and long before I had assimilated them into my thought and behavior patterns. Years would pass before I would give them my own more mature interpretation and elaboration. I had not yet learned from my own personal experience that we can, by our own efforts and with appropriate professional assistance and guidance, change what appears to be an inexorably dismal fate to a fate more of one's choosing. Indeed, this is the encapsulated message of this book.

At the time I formulated my future case histories, I had not yet learned the above message. My error in thinking about the three of us was, in effect, to think about us as though we were automobiles. Although from different assembly lines, each automobile was appropriately equipped with the prototypic parts, such as the carburetor, the distributor, the alternator, the drive-shaft, and so on. My problem, from this naive viewpoint, was that I had been given a lemon. What I overlooked was that the human, unlike the car, has the inherent capacity for self-regulation, self-repair, regeneration, preventive maintenance, and upgrading to a better model.

WHAT IS NORMAL?

I'd like to add that the error in my thinking was not mine alone. I had merely joined in the "consensus trance."[9] The same kinds of assumptions I made with my future case histories still underlie much of clinical practice. Despite knowledge to the contrary, the tendency toward homogenization of patients persists in medical care. Nowhere is this better reflected than in the periodic medical checkup. This health assessment usually includes a thorough physical examination and assorted laboratory tests, analyses, and measurements. The purpose is to obtain the concentrations of various components of the blood and other body fluids as well as measures of other physiological and biochemical parameters. The numbers are then compared with those said to be the normal values. Each item for a given patient is declared to be either within normal limits or above or below normal limits, usually hyper- or hypo-something. From previous experiences, we all know that deviation from normal limits probably requires some remedial action or at least careful watching.

What is at issue here is not the value of periodic checkups. They are certainly important in the detection of early signs of disease or threatening functional impairments. What is at issue is the concept of normal. Overlooked is the fact that just as there is an infinite variety of ways of being human, so is there an infinite variety of ways of being normal. Also forgotten is that the so-called normal range for each item is based on the average of the values found in a large number of individuals who are apparently free of disease. Do we know that the averages for all the measured items are indeed desirable for every person? Is it not likely that different people, according to who they are, what they do, how they live, and their ages, require different combinations of numbers that are uniquely normal for them?

In 1956, Roger J. Williams, PhD, a distinguished biochemist and nutritionist, published a book that deals brilliantly with this issue, titled *Biochemical Individuality*.[10] In this book, he reviews studies by himself, his collaborators, and many other accomplished investigators. The results present the range of differences among humans who are apparently in good health with respect to such items as composition of the body fluids, enzymic patterns, endocrine activities, excretion patterns, metabolism, nutritional needs, body composition, size of various organs, sensory thresholds, and so on. Differences of 30 to 600 percent were common among individual items, and even twentyfold (2,000 percent) differences were found! Dr. Williams calculated that given the concentration of nineteen substances in the blood, there was only one chance in a half million of being in the middle, 50 percent range with respect to all nineteen items. In other words and paradoxically, deviations from normal are perfectly normal!

One can envision studies on two different hypothetical groups of healthy young men. Young men, apparently free of disease and usually students, have historically been the favored subjects in the quest for normal values, a bias in and of itself. In this hypothetical cohort of subjects, let us choose ten young men who are very uniform with respect to age, body build, weight and size, occupation, activities, diet, habits, and so on, and in another group choose ten young men who are very diverse with respect to the same features. Although the two groups could have similar or even identical averages for each of the measured items, the assortment of future clinical problems and levels of health in the two groups would most likely be very different. It is also likely that the physiological paths and future case histories within the second group would be more divergent.

In other words, there is such an endless variety of ways of being normal that the whole concept of normality becomes nebulous and arbitrary. Like the concept of the heart and the liver, normal is a concept made up by humans and not a phenomenon occurring in nature. The question remains, however, "How do the different ways of being human (and normal) relate to current and future health?" Unfortunately, while work like that of Dr. Williams's has had a significant impact on the discipline of anthropology, it has had negligible influence on medical education, research, or practice. In a paper presented at a meeting of the National Academy of Sciences in 1955, Dr. Williams declared, "If we think that a typical human population consists of individuals who are 'about average' in most respects, our thinking is bound to be unrealistic and futile, because a typical population contains no such individuals." He urged that the "statistical man" must be "dethroned from his position as the center of our interest" for he has no counterpart in a population of real individuals.[11] Incidentally, Roger Williams died in 1988 at the age of ninety-four—active, enthusiastic, and productive to the very end.

The concept of normal becomes even more nebulous when applied in geriatric practice. Nobody knows what is normal for people in their fifties, sixties, seventies, or eighties since nobody knows which of the differences from healthy young men and women are intrinsic to the aging process, which are genetic, and which are due to extrinsic factors subsumed under lifestyle and history.[12] We remain largely in the dark, therefore, about which departures from normal are appropriate and even essential in the older person and which are signs of incipient or existing illness.

HEALTH AND THE BIOLOGY OF HUMAN VARIATION

I was primed for such concepts as these by Dr. Williams from my exposure to the ambient emphasis at the Kirksville College of Osteopathic Medicine on treating the person, the whole person and not merely the ailment and affected organ, and by my interest in differences in human vulnerability, awakened by my observations on the first few freshman classes I taught at the college. Later, my own transformation gave added meaning and emotional impetus to this interest. Thus it was that I discovered the discipline of medical anthropology, exemplified by two provocative symposia sponsored in the 1960s by the New York Academy of Sciences.[13]

At that point, I became more and more convinced that this was the area in which the future of medicine lay as I fully realized that its future could not merely be in the continued quest for individual causes or risk factors of disease or for its cure. The future, I firmly believe, lies in the study of the biology of human variation in relation to levels of health, vulnerability, susceptibilities, and longevity.

Even the well-established causes of diseases become causes only when permitted by other factors in the individual's life. For example, only a minority (apparently a small minority) of veteran heavy smokers fall victim to lung cancer. This does not by any means diminish the crucial importance of smoking as a *risk factor* (a much better concept than cause), but it does mean that other personal factors or combinations of factors can determine how risky such risk factors are. Obviously, favorable combinations of personal factors are the causes of noncancer, of nondisease, and of health, to which medical research and practice must give increasing attention.

This principle has been dramatically demonstrated in the world-wide struggle against the AIDS epidemic. Although the human immunodeficiency virus (HIV) has long been identified as the cause of AIDS, multinational research efforts to find or develop a cure or an effective vaccine to disarm or destroy the virus have been unsuccessful. General disappointment and frustration were evident at the Tenth International Conference on AIDS held in Yokohama, Japan, in August 1994.[14]

One encouraging note was sounded, however, in an address given by Dr. Jay A. Levy of the University of California at San Francisco, who is a distinguished veteran AIDS researcher. He said that, given the lack of a cure or vaccine, the research emphasis should turn to slowing the pace at which HIV infection develops into the deadly disease. He urged the researchers to focus on long-term survivors, some of whom have been HIV-positive for sixteen years, because "They're telling us a lot about *what the human body can do*" (emphasis added). In short, he suggested that we begin to study the causes of nondisease, of non-AIDS, and of health.[15]

The more that research and practice can turn from a focus on specific causative factors in diseases to the anti–risk factors in healthy individuals, the better equipped we will be for health enhancement and disease prevention both nationwide and, ultimately, worldwide. This new focus should by no means ignore or deemphasize differences in genetic endowments; they are undeniably of great and often critical importance. The new focus is meant to emphasize the objective of making the most of our inheritance and of moderating or even nullifying genetic predispositions.

The longer that medicine and medical education delay expanding their attention to the study of health and its enhancement as the most comprehensive approach to disease prevention, and the longer that they remain so absorbed in the high-tech treatment of after-the-fact, late-stage, and terminal disease, then the longer chronic degenerative diseases will continue to flourish. Meanwhile, the only option for individuals is for them to take charge of their own preventive maintenance and their own upgrading. Further, those individuals should seek out professional care that supports these kinds of proactive objectives.

Having lived as long as I have, I have had the opportunity to observe at close range the individual and divergent paths of many of my contemporaries, be they friends, relatives, or colleagues. I have also had to observe their denouements. A few of my contemporaries who are close to my age are still in vibrant health, still fully and rewardingly engaged. Some even compete in demanding athletic events, such as triathlons. At the other extreme, there are those, including many of my former students, whose lives have at various ages been severely circumscribed or prematurely terminated by chronic disease and disabilities.

I have many sad memories of friends, fellow scientists, and faculty members in the latter group. Through the years, I visited many of them in hospitals, sickrooms, and nursing homes. I listened to concerns about their families, interrupted work, and work that would never be finished. I discussed their clinical futures with them. I wept with those who knew that recovery was impossible and with those who knew that death was imminent. Lost forever are the further contributions they were prepared to make to literature, art, science, education, and the enlightenment and welfare of others. I attended the funerals and memorial services of many and helped carry some to their graves.

As I bring the image of each of these cherished and admired friends and colleagues to mind and am once again touched by sadness, a recurrent and persistent question thrusts itself into my consciousness (and conscience): Had I had the opportunity and the requisite wisdom at the time, what would I have said long before disaster struck that might have helped each move toward a path that would have led to a happier outcome? Meanwhile, what lessons from my own experience, that of other healthy old people, as well as from published research that can now be conveyed to others so that they may test them in their own lives?

In this chapter, I have challenged the concept of *normal* and made the case for studying the causes of health, not disease, within the context of individual lives. In the next chapter, we will explore the mythology of health and disease and its contribution to the origins of human vulnerability.

NOTES

1. H. Brody, *Stories of Sickness* (New York: Oxford University Press, 2003).

2. Department of Health and Human Services, "Healthy People 2010," http://www.healthypeople.gov (accessed March 1, 2007).

3. C. A. Depp and D. V. Jeste, "Definitions and Predictors of Successful Aging: A Comprehensive Review of Larger Quantitative Studies," *American Journal Geriatric Psychiatry* 14 (2006): 6–20.

4. N. M. Peel, R. J. McClure, and H. P. Bartlett, "Behavioral Determinants of Healthy Aging," *American Journal of Preventive Medicine* 28 (2005): 298–304; M. von Faber et al., "Successful Aging in the Oldest Old: Who Can Be Characterized as Successfully Aged?" *Archives of Internal Medicine* 161 (2001): 2694–2700.

5. S. G. Leveille et al., "Aging Successfully until Death in Old Age: Opportunities for Increasing Active Life Expectancy," *American Journal of Epidemiology* 149 (1999): 654–64; A. B. Newman et al., "'Successful Aging': Effect of Subclinical Cardiovascular Disease," *Archives of Internal Medicine* 163 (2003): 2315–22; W. J. Strawbridge et al., "Successful Aging: Predictors and Associated Activities," *American Journal of Epidemiology* 144 (1996): 135–41.

6. G. W. Duff, "Evidence for Genetic Variation as a Factor in Maintaining Health," *American Journal of Clinical Nutrition* 83 (2006): 431S–435S.

7. T. Seeman and X. Chen, "Risk and Protective Factors for Physical Functioning in Older Adults with and without Chronic Conditions: Macarthur Studies of Successful Aging," *Journals of Gerontology, Series B Psychological Sciences and Social Sciences* 57 (2002): S135–S144.

8. R. J. Hodes, V. Cahan, and M. Pruzan, "The National Institute on Aging at Its Twentieth Anniversary: Achievements and Promise of Research on Aging," *Journal of the American Geriatrics Society* 44 (1996): 204–206.

9. C. Tart, *Waking Up* (Boston: Shambhala, 1986).

10. R. J. Williams, *Biochemical Individuality* (New York: Wiley, 1956).

11. R. J. Williams, "Biochemical Approach to the Study of Personality," *Psychiatric Research Reports* (December 1955): 31–33.

12. S. J. Glatt et al., "Successful Aging: From Phenotype to Genotype," *Biological Psychiatry* 62, no. 4 (2007): 282–93.

13. S. H. Posinsky, *Medicine and Anthropology: The New York Academy of Medicine Lectures to the Laity*, no. 20, ed. I. Galdston (New York: International Universities Press, 1960).

14. P. B. Berger, "New Directions in Research: Report from the Tenth International Conference on AIDS," *Canadian Medical Association Journal* 152 (1995): 1991–95.

15. Ibid.

Chapter 7

THE MYTHOLOGY OF
HEALTH AND DISEASE

"Enlightenment comes on its own and unexpectedly when I cease to
pursue it."

—I. M. Korr

The next three chapters are concerned with those features peculiar
to the human species and human life that render us uniquely vulnerable to illness and infirmity, and even to extinction. Together, they
render us "The Fragile Species" that Lewis Thomas described in a
wise and charming book of that title.[1]

Some of these human features are natural concomitants of our biological evolution. They are subject to change in the course of any further evolution.[2] Others, much more hazardous to our health and even
threatening to the very survival of the human race, are artifacts and by-
products of our cultural evolution and our civilizations.[3] Fortunately,
just as these hazards have been created by humans, so too can they be
mitigated and even eliminated by our deliberate individual and collective effort.

Among these man-made hazards are half-truths and even total
falsehoods that we have made up about health, illness, and aging;

some have become our most widely shared and largely unchallenged beliefs. Their hazard is in the degree to which they shape our behavior, policies, and practices. These pervasive myths are part of what psychologist Charles Tart characterized as the "consensus trance" in which most of us live our lives.[4] We do not ordinarily question much or consider that there may be other and possibly better ways of thinking and behaving with respect to health, disease, and aging.

In this chapter, I will identify some of these unspoken and unquestioned beliefs. I will also offer some alternatives based on the perspectives discussed in part 2 on the four guiding principles. I am convinced that the consensus trance in the realm of health and illness leads millions of Americans, young and old, to accept lower levels of health, higher levels of morbidity, a poorer quality of life, and shorter lives than are within their reach.

Along with the pollution of our air, water, soil, and food as well as poverty, ignorance, racism, and other forms of discrimination, such shared misconceptions are a serious impediment to the improvement of our national health. Collectively these cause the health of this great nation, despite its superb medical technology and its immense investment in healthcare, to continue to compare unfavorably, by our own criteria, with other advanced and even not-so-advanced nations. See, for example, *The Betrayal of Health* by Joseph D. Beasley, MD, for further elaboration of my point.[5]

Although the guiding principles discussed in part 2 are hardly new and may even seem self-evident, they are in many ways, nevertheless, in conflict with prevailing notions about health and illness. They tend to not be assimilated into our thinking and are incorporated even less into personal and professional health practices or public policies.

What follows are a few of the myths and misconceptions that dramatically impact our healthcare as I have come to perceive them. I have also included a discussion of the corrections that I believe are needed. To quote humorist and philosopher Josh Billings, "It ain't what a man don't know that makes him a fool; it's the things he does know that ain't so."[6] (See figure 1 in the photo insert.)

MYTH 1: HEALTH VERSUS DISEASE

Health is defined in the World Health Organization's constitution as "a state of complete physical, mental and social well-being and not merely the absence of disease or infirmity."[7] This is perhaps the most widely quoted definition of health and, at the same time, the most ignored in thought and practice.

How, for example, do professionals in the field of public health assess and compare the health of nations, communities, or other populations? By assessing well-being? No, they assess public health by means of morbidity and mortality tables. In other words, by disease and death rates! In short, they measure the incidence of various diseases and the numbers of deaths due to those diseases; these numbers are then regarded as the indices of a nation's health. Based on the collection of this information, it would seem that public health professionals are more concerned with the postponement of death than with the quality of life as defined by physical, mental, and social well-being.

As humans, we grow up in our society with the unarticulated belief that each of us at a given time is in either of two states: either we are sick, or we are well. Further, if we are not sick, then we are considered well and, therefore, not candidates for healthcare. After all, healthy people don't have health problems and have nothing to cure. Thus, at one moment we regard ourselves as healthy, and the next moment, having caught a cold or the flu, having experienced the first anginal attack or ulcer pain, we cross an imaginary threshold into illness and eligibility for healthcare. This myth of health versus illness is so insidious (and I will admit I was slow to recognize it) that I was well into my forties before I learned that one can be free of identifiable disease but still be in poor health and lacking in well-being. In short, there are gradations of health.

This is not, however, just a lay misconception. Most physicians have graduated from medical school with a similar dichotomous belief, whether it was explicitly taught or inferred from observation of their teacher models. Medical education, like medical practice, is dedicated to the care of sick and injured people; there is little reason or opportunity to learn about health and its enhancement.

For the physician, unfortunately, health enhancement lacks the drama, the heroics, the magic, or the financial rewards of miracle cures. That responsibility has been left to others by default. There are, however, encouraging signs of growing professional awareness that perhaps the promotion of health may be within the province of what purports to be a healthcare system if only for the reason that it has value in the prevention of disease. (Unfortunately, little encouragement comes from insurers, either governmental or private, who provide negligible if any coverage for preventive measures, much less health enhancement.)

The truth is that there is no boundary, no threshold between health and disease, illness and wellness, the normal and the pathological. Health and disease are linked in an uninterrupted continuum, a sort of spectrum, if you will, that extends from high-level health at one end, through progressively lower levels of health, and then to various degrees of illness until it reaches terminal disease at the other end. At any moment, each of us is at some band on the spectrum and moving in one direction or the other. The choices we make (or are given) in the way we live are crucial determinants of our position on the spectrum and of the direction in which we move. *Just remember, we always have the opportunity to move to a brighter hue.*

Unfortunately, because the focus of medicine and of medical education and research is on the disease end of the spectrum rather than on health and its enhancement, only a minute portion of the nation's health bill is truly for prevention of disease and promotion of health. More and more of the nation's healthcare costs are slated for the expensive, high-technology, and long-term care of those who are chronically ill and dying. As important and necessary as those costs are, however, they cannot produce healthier people. That remains the responsibility of individuals who are given the requisite knowledge, means, and propitious environments.

Despite this, doctors and others can remove obstacles from the path toward high-level health, and they may be able guide us in the choices we make. But it is we who make the choices and we who do the moving. To assume that we are experiencing good health because we have not crossed the dreaded threshold into illness is to deny ourselves the opportunity to enjoy progressively higher levels of well-being.

What can one expect to enjoy at these higher levels? One benefit, obviously, is relative freedom from disease, for the healthier we are, the less vulnerable we are to unfavorable circumstances and environments in our lives and the less likely we are to become ill. Indeed, one of the benefits of health enhancement is that it is the most comprehensive and the most effective form of preventive medicine. Welcome as it is, the preventive value is only a by-product. The primary benefits of high-level wellness, as I learned from my own personal experience, are (1) that it is empowering and (2) that it feels good.

I have difficulty explaining what I mean by feeling good. Although we seem to recognize it in others, it really must be experienced. I go to sleep each night and wake each morning looking forward to the new day and the tasks, challenges, pleasures, surprises, and new learning opportunities that the day will bring. I take pleasure in the things I get done and in their doing; I look forward to the things yet to be done. As much as I enjoy being with those I love, I am renewed each day during my alone time. My joy in living communicates itself to others, and it also brings them pleasure, which doubles mine. My joy seems to be felt by every cell in my body, and I, in turn, feel energized and empowered. By empowered, I mean that high-level health increases the potential and multiplies the possibilities for living fully, vigorously, actively, enthusiastically, productively, and joyfully.

Halbert L. Dunn, MD, PhD, a former chief of the National Office of Vital Statistics, a division within the United States Public Health Service, first described "high-level wellness" (a term he coined). Having recently rediscovered this idea among his writings as I prepared this book, it struck me as an eloquent elaboration of my concept of empowerment and feeling good. He stated:

Nothing is cherished quite so much by you and me as this thing we call good health. We both know that good health means far more than just not being ill. It also means an awareness and aliveness to the world in which we live.

When all is right within me, my body well, and my thoughts in tune with the world, every sense organ opens to drink in the joys of all I see and feel and hear. I am intoxicated at such times with the ecstasy of being alive. No task is too difficult, no hurdle too high. That is good health in this world of mine. At least, it is a major part of health! Of that I'm sure. It is the difference between *existing* and *living*. It cannot be unless my thoughts are right. I sometimes wonder when I feel this way if a disease bug, knocking for entrance, does not find himself overwhelmed by the power-drunk blood cells in my body. He must at least have a battle on his hands.

And of another thing I am sure. This feeling of aliveness when it is mine spreads like the rising sun into the world about me. You respond to it in me as I do in you. A song comes to your lips unasked. A pleasant glow warms your thoughts.[8]

In a more objective, less rhapsodic mood, Dr. Dunn distinguished high-level wellness from good health, which he felt, as I do, had come to mean merely a passive state of "absence of disease or infirmity."[9] In my opinion, however, which I expressed to him many years ago, the need is not to create a new term but to redefine health. By doing so and in such a manner as to remind us that health is derived from the same stem as *whole*, we can by definition denote the total intactness of the person.

In the same book, Dr. Dunn describes wellness (for which I substitute health) not as a state but as process that is (1) a direction of progress toward higher potentials of functioning (or in my earlier metaphor toward brighter hues on the health spectrum), (2) a continual challenge to live at a fuller potential, and (3) the integration of the total individual in body, mind, and spirit in the functioning process. Dr. Dunn goes on to explain, "The term 'spirit' in this context is not used in a metaphysical sense but rather in the sense of a 'zone of interaction' between body and mind." From this viewpoint, health is a continual process of growth, of becoming, of enlarging potentials, and of continually unfolding horizons. This is a viewpoint I share.

It is sad that, despite our medical knowledge and technology, so few in our society experience optimal health as a way of life. It is especially sad when one realizes that to have that experience, one need only live in such a way as to empower the "physician within" by "living in harmony with nature's laws," as Hippocrates put it almost twenty-four centuries ago.[10]

MYTH 2: CROSSING ANOTHER THRESHOLD AND THE DISEASES OF AGING

In the spring of 1974, two or three months before my sixty-fifth birthday, I received a postcard from the federal Social Security Agency instructing me to appear at the local branch office in order to file my application for Medicare insurance. I shall never forget the emotional shock that I experienced, the depression that followed, or the humiliation I shared with the other older people who also waited in the office, resignedly, for some sign of acknowledgment from the clerks whose ages averaged about one-third of ours. Though still in excellent health, still professionally and athletically active, and still able to play a vigorous game of tennis against able players many years younger, I had, despite my training and experience as a medical researcher and educator, bought into an absurd health-related myth.

I had unconsciously come to assume that on my sixty-fifth birthday, I would cross the dreaded threshold into senior citizenship, which marked the beginning of the "Great Decline." The knowledge that the cost of my diseases of aging would be substantially defrayed by my fellow taxpayers brought little comfort at the time. Fortunately, I had learned enough during the preceding twenty-five years about health and disease that I was soon able to laugh at the absurdity of the myth and at my own ludicrous, unconscious, and unquestioning acceptance of it. On this issue, I too had been living in a consensus trance. At the time of this writing, though all the appropriate natural physiological and psychological changes of further maturing have occurred, the decline into disease and dependency has yet to begin.

To clarify, the myth to which I had uncritically given credence was that aging is a period of progressive deterioration, that increasing disability and the diseases of aging are the inevitable products of the aging process, and that aging is itself pathological.

In the first place, age sixty-five does not mark transition into old age or anything else other than eligibility for federal subsidies. That age was chosen arbitrarily and in response to a precedent said to have been set by Chancellor Bismarck of Germany in 1889.[11] In seeking an appropriate age for military pensions to start, the story goes, the chancellor began with what was then the life expectancy, forty-three years, and added for no apparent logical reason half that number so that he arrived at age sixty-five. Were we to apply the same formula today for the calculation of retirement benefits, the pensionable age would be about one hundred and twelve!

Second, regardless of when old age is said to begin, the disabling conditions and diseases of older people are not inherent in the aging process. With the possible exception of those diseases that are related to genetic or congenital defects or predispositions, the chronic illnesses that are so common among the elderly are largely the products of ways of living and of circumstances that are insufficiently supportive of the physiological and biochemical processes discussed in preceding chapters. Speaking metaphorically, the so-called diseases of aging are ascribable to the deteriorated competence of the physician within brought on by neglect, abuse, and the imposition of deleterious living conditions. Hence, the chronic infirmities and diseases of old age are created mainly by us humans. They are, therefore, largely preventable through the adoption of lifestyles and living conditions that support the physician within.

Since we are mortal with a finite life span however favorable our life circumstances, ultimate fatal exhaustion and failure of the circulation and other bodily functions is a fact of life. The object, as James F.

Fries, MD, has written, is to delay and "compress" morbidity into the latest possible moments of life.[12]

If the health problems of the elderly are not an intrinsic aspect of growing older, why then are they so much more common among the older population than the younger population? I think the answer lies in the same reason that, given time, dripping water can wear away rock or the porcelain in a sink. The longer we live, the greater the opportunity for minor defects or impediments, which may in themselves produce no symptoms or disabilities, to take their toll; the greater the opportunity to involve more and more organs and physiological processes in ever-widening circles of chronic dysfunction. You can begin to see the importance of living in such ways and in such circumstances as to minimize those seemingly innocuous but erosive drips.

Why don't people choose to live in these more healthful ways even when they have the option and the means to make that choice? As it must be evident to the reader by now, I am convinced that major factors are (1) the widely held belief that infirmity and lost mobility are the unavoidable price of long life and (2) the expectation that by the time chronic illness has developed, a cure will have been discovered. (See Myth 4.)

It is no wonder that decrepitude and impaired mobility have been painted into the stereotypic image we have of the aged as frail, fragile, stooped, stiff, shuffling, sedentary, sexless, self-absorbed, dependent, and joyless humans. Having grown up with that image as the norm, aging people often tend to conform to what is culturally expected of them. Ironically, the youthful old person is looked upon as an aberration, a departure from what is natural. In truth, it is the young-old person who is the natural product, with the stereotype being the man-made artifact.

MYTH 3: REST AS REWARD

The preceding stereotype is reinforced by our widespread policy of retirement at some arbitrary age. In effect, we say, "Look, having worked all your life, you've now earned your rest. Go now, and enjoy your reward." Reward? The cost of withdrawal from active, contributory life and its challenges is enormous in terms of lost mobility, health, and joy of living. It also has an enormous economic impact by limiting future independence and productivity. The effects of prolonged inactivity, lost mobility, and the generalized atrophy of disuse (chapter 3) conventionally attributed to aging itself can be reproduced experimentally in young people by enforced long-term inactivity.[13] For too many, this reward is a cruel punishment, producing tragic results.

Life is for living, not for vacating. Rest will come soon enough and last an eternity. The well-known image from nineteenth-century American painter James McNeill Whistler of his mother in her rocking chair needs to be changed.[14] In other words, Grandma and Grandpa need to get off their rockers.

MYTH 4: THE HEALTHCARE SYSTEM IS THE SOURCE OF HEALTH

This myth, long familiar to me, was poignantly dramatized for me in the fall of 1985. A local agency was conducting a series of Saturday morning seminars for pre-retirement employees of various companies, institutions, and organizations in town; all attendees held important positions and were well educated. The theme of the series was "Preparing for Retirement." In one seminar, I was the second of two speakers, the first being a banker lecturing on the subject of financial security. My topic was health in the retirement years.

I began by commending the group for their foresightedness in planning well in advance of their retirement for their financial security. "Now," I asked, "what are you doing to ensure that you will get to enjoy that security in good health and for as long as possible?"

"Oh, we have that covered too," was the rather smug reply.

"How?" I persisted.

The answer came quickly: "We have health insurance."

This, it seems to me, is the most seductive misconception of all:

the idea that physicians, medicines, hospitals, medical technology, and the healthcare system can impart health. The truth is that no person or persons, whatever their knowledge and skills, whatever the available technology and resources, can impart health to another person any more than they can impart character, charm, wit, intelligence, integrity, or any other desirable human trait. Health cannot be transfused like blood or transplanted like a kidney.

The physician and the treatment may help, maybe even crucially, but they cannot restore or maintain our health for us. Only we can do this for ourselves with our own natural resources. This is the meaning of personal responsibility for health. Again, this is by no means to downplay the physician's role but to "up-play" the patient's role in his or her recovery from illness and in the maintenance and improvement of his or her health. I would like to point out that this notion has important implications for the patient-doctor relationship. When a patient becomes a proactive participant of healthy living, the patient-doctor relationship becomes a partnership rather than a relationship between an authoritarian figure and a compliant one. (Nothing frustrates physicians more than the noncompliant patient who does not follow orders.)

On occasions when I have overheard a physician say with justifiable pride in a patient's improvement that "I cured that patient," a ludicrous image comes to mind: a music lover in his home who selects a favorite recording from his collection, inserts it into his CD player, flips a switch or two, adjusts a dial or two, then leans back in his armchair, saying, "What beautiful music I play." The music I refer to above came not from the doctor's prescription, syringe, or scalpel but from within the patient. At best, the physician's treatment allowed it to be heard, and I will concede that this is no small contribution.

So the principle of this discussion applies even if we use the conventional measures of health. Remember those morbidity and mortality figures? Let us consider the so-called conquest of the major infectious diseases and devastating epidemics, such as tuberculosis, plague, smallpox, and cholera, which underlie the large increase in life expectancy of last century. These were not, with the likely exception

of polio, conquests. That is, they were not the effects of medical interventions. As has been shown by epidemiologists, historians, and
others, the incidence and severity of these diseases had begun to
decline long before, maybe even centuries before, any effective medical interventions, such as vaccines and antibiotics, were available.[15]
The declines (see appendix 1) were due to such nonmedical factors as
improved living, working, and housing conditions; better and cleaner
food; sanitation; sewerage; launderable undergarments; purer water;
pasteurized milk; and the waning virulence of some of the "bugs." For
the most part, sulfa drugs, antibiotics, and vaccines were responsible
only for deepening the downward slopes and the final coup de grâce.

Perhaps the ultimate absurdity emanating from the pretense that
the healthcare system is the purveyor of health was the proposed and
rejected legislation to establish federal catastrophic health insurance.
Presumably, this insurance was meant to protect the elderly against a
threatening epidemic of catastrophic health!

MYTH 5: DISEASES AS AUTONOMOUS THINGS

Also included in our consensus trance are the commonly shared views
about the nature of diseases. Our very language reflects the myths we
have unwittingly come to accept. We speak of diseases like they were
autonomous entities, predatory in nature, always hovering and
awaiting the opportunity to attack. For example, we speak and write,
even in professional circles, of the natural history of disease as though
it were a free-living organism. Physicians argue as to whether a pattern of manifestation represents a real entity, as though it were a
species of flora or fauna. We speak of fighting disease and of
increasing resistance to disease as though it were indeed a predator
threatening from without. The question that immediately comes to
mind is, where is the disease while it is being resisted?

"The disease has run its course" is offered as the explanation for
the recovery from, say, an acute infectious disease, as though the

course had been run on an inanimate terrain. One hears doctors and even teachers of doctors say, rather sanctimoniously, that the physician must treat the patient as well as the disease as if it were possible to treat the disease in any way other than by treating the patient![16]

The fact is that nobody has ever seen a disease. All that one can see are persons who are ill in various, more or less, patterned ways. There is some basis in the satirical comment that the patient goes to the doctor with an illness and leaves with a disease. Despite the talk about multiple factors in every disease, there is the common notion that every disease, whether it is cancer, heart disease, rheumatoid arthritis, or any other, has *a* cause and *a* cure, both usually awaiting discovery. In our quest, we continue to overlook the human, personal factors that permit the so-called causes to become causes and the cures to be cures. That is, the participation of the patient in the pathogenesis (causation) and in the recovery is slighted. We blame the cause for the disease and credit the doctor for the cure.

To Louis Pasteur's credit, late in his distinguished career, he pointed out the error of this view. He even went so far as to challenge this view in infectious diseases where specific causes were known. He stated that the "terrain" provided by the patient is crucial and that when the bacteria have proliferated in the patient's body, there must have been a preexisting illness that rendered the "host" hospitable to the bacteria.[17]

A corollary myth is that every disease has an affinity for a particular part of the body or a specific process, and that spot is the site of the disease. Thus, we have diseases of the skin, kidneys, lungs, digestion, metabolism, and so forth. Appropriate treatment of the organ or process will, according to this view, restore the patient to health. There is no denying that the patient with an ulcer of the duodenum, for example, is in pain and distress, or that appropriate treatment directed to the duodenum will bring relief. The fact is, however, that the patient is not ill because he has an ulcer; he has an ulcer because he is not well, providing a terrain in which the physiological processes inevitably culminate in peptic ulcer. Of course, the terrain is determined by all the factors and circumstances in that person's life, past and present, as previously discussed.

In view of the functional interlocking of all the body parts and the oneness of bodymind, the concept that disease is contained in this or that organ or tissue, which then becomes the target of treatment, is as insupportable as the preceding myths. To conceive of my previous example, the duodenal ulcer, as a gastroenterological entity due to hypersecretion and hypermotility of the small intestine is as nonsensical as calling the tears of the bereaved an ophthalmologic entity due to hypersecretion by the tear glands. The ulcer patient is also weeping but through another part of his body.

Thus, illness is not that of the organ but of the person; the organ is simply a victim of what ails the patient and of the internal environment in which it functions. The organ is neither the site nor the source of the ailment.[18] Healing of the part awaits healing of the person. By analogy, silencing the squeaking wheel with a shot of grease may address the complaint of the owner-driver, but it overlooks the fact that the wheel squeaks because the entire car may be out of line, carelessly driven into curbs, exposed to corrosive agents, or poorly maintained. The grease does not solve the problem and invites the squeaks of other parts.

A RECAPITULATION

1. Health is not merely the absence of disease. Health occurs in a wide range of levels, extending on a continuous spectrum from high levels of well-being through lower levels and on to minor and major illness through to life-endangering and terminal disease.
2. No person can be made well or healthy by another. The available skills and technology, helpful and supportive though they may be, are not a substitute for the person's own physician within. The recovery, maintenance, and enhancement of health ultimately depend on the resources within each individual. Hence,

the care and nurturing of those resources by each individual, as well as the preparation that enables the individual to assume that responsibility as effectively as possible, is critical.

3. Infirmity and decrepitude are not the inevitable products of aging but of lifestyles and circumstances that do not favor higher levels of health. That is, individual behaviors that have not been sufficiently supportive of the indwelling health maintenance organization are counter to optimum health.

4. Inactivity and withdrawal from the challenges of active living are major contributors to illness and immobility in the elderly. The disuse of bodymind is detrimental to one's health.

5. Diseases are not things that attack from without. They are processes within the body and are the result of responses of the person to unfavorable circumstances both within and of his or her life.

In the next chapter, we will examine as a source of human vulnerability our biological machinery and its adaptation to the world we have created.

NOTES

1. L. Thomas, *The Fragile Species* (New York: Scribner, 1992).

2. E. J. Larson, *Evolution* (New York: Random House, 2004).

3. R. M. Nesse and G. C. Williams, *Why We Get Sick: The New Science of Darwinian Medicine* (New York: Vintage, 1994).

4. C. Tart, *Waking Up* (Boston: Shambhala, 1986).

5. J. D. Beasley, *The Betrayal of Health* (New York: Times Books, 1991).

6. J. Billings, *Josh Billings, Hiz Sayings* (Kila, MT: Kessinger, 2006).

7. World Health Organization, "About WHO," 2007, http://www.who .int/about/en/ (accessed February 28, 2007).

8. H. L. Dunn, *Your World and Mine*, 2nd ed. (New York: Exposition Press, 1956), p. 25.

9. H. L. Dunn, *High-Level Wellness* (Arlington, VA: R. W. Beatty, 1961).

10. M. J. Schiefsky, trans., *Hippocrates on Ancient Medicine* (New York: Brill, 2005).

11. Social Security Online, "History Archives," 2007, http://www.ssa.gov/history/archives/archives.html (accessed February 28, 2007).

12. J. F. Fries, "Aging, Illness, and Health Policy: Implications of the Compression of Morbidity," *Perspectives in Biology and Medicine* 31 (1988): 407–28.

13. D. Paddon-Jones et al., "Atrophy and Impaired Muscle Protein Synthesis during Prolonged Inactivity and Stress," *Journal of Clinical Endocrinology and Metabolism* 91 (2006): 4836–41.

14. "Whistler, James Abbott McNeill," WebMuseum, Paris, http://www.ibiblio.org/wm/paint/auth/whistler/ (accessed March 28, 2007).

15. R. Dubos, *Mirage of Health: Utopias, Progress and Biological Change* (New York: Harper, 1959); T. McKeown, *The Role of Medicine: Dream, Mirage, or Nemesis?* (London: Nuffield Provincial Hospital Trust, 1976).

16. I. M. Korr, "Medical Education: The Resistance to Change," *Advances* 4 (1987): 5–10.

17. L. Pasteur and J. Lister, *Germ Theory and Its Application to Medicine & on the Antiseptic Principle of the Practice of Surgery* (Amherst, NY: Prometheus Books, 1996).

18. S. B. Nuland, *The Wisdom of the Body* (New York: Knopf, 1997).

Chapter 8

OLD MACHINERY IN
NEW CONTEXTS

"The sharper my view of now, the further I can see ahead."

—I. M. Korr

HUMANS AND HUMAN HEALTH
AND ILLNESS AS PRODUCTS OF EVOLUTION

This chapter and the one that follows continue the examination of those factors peculiar to the human species that influence our potential for health and our susceptibility to illness. Experience—mine and that of countless others—has convinced me that the more we appreciate the unique features of human biology and their variations from person to person, the more we are enabled to adopt health as a way of life. And more important, as a way of a long and fulfilling life.

The development of comprehensive and productive approaches to these issues requires appreciation of the human race as a product of evolution, closely related to other mammals and most particularly to other primates.[1] You might ask what human evolution has to do with human health and illness. As we shall see, our attainable levels of health and our susceptibility to various infirmities are as much the products of evolution, both biological and cultural, as we are.[2]

OUR HAND-ME-DOWN BIOLOGICAL MACHINERY

The fact is that we have inherited from our ancestors all of our biological machinery, such as our cells, tissues, organs, and systems as well as the multitude of processes going on within them and in which they participate. These things have evolved over millions upon millions of years, progressively becoming more efficient and refined in their operations and in their service to the total organism.[3] To be sure, there has been, in the emergence of humans, considerable rearrangement as well as some modification and elaboration that has most notably occurred in the nervous system.[4] However, the same components and the same chemical, metabolic, genetic, physiological, and other processes are recognizable in all mammalian species whether they be human, feline, canine, equine, or rodent. These processes are apparent even in lower vertebrates. Indeed and as has been stated previously, most of our knowledge about fundamental human biology has been acquired from the study of lower animals. Even the study of single-celled amoebae, worms, insects, and marine snails has added to our knowledge.

Included in the hand-me-down biological apparatus of humans are all those wonderful defensive, reparative, regenerative, regulatory, healing, immune, and detoxifying mechanisms that make up the *vis medicatrix naturae*, or the inner healthcare system. These mechanisms survived and continued to develop in the course of millions of years of evolution because they worked. Let me add that they continue to serve humans very well today when we let them. After all, they are the source of our potential for optimal health.

Where are the biological differences between humans and other animal species with which humankind shares its fundamental components and mechanisms? The difference is in the interactive unity, that environmental context I discussed in chapter 2. The biological machinery that now serves humans evolved under conditions, like those found in the ancient seas, rivers, lakes, soil, jungles, caves, forests, and deserts, which were vastly different from what exists in modern times.[5] That inherited biological machinery, while not fundamentally changed, is now called upon to serve different kinds of organisms, living totally different lives in vastly different environments. What is more, those environments include not only those provided by nature but those created by humans. As we know, our man-made environments are subject to endless and rapid transformations, some of which are detrimental to our health and the very survival of ourselves and other species.

OLD PARTS IN A NEW TOTALITY

In what ways does the human context in which our body components operate differ from that of, for example, our most closely related species? The first, most conspicuous, and perhaps most important difference is our upright, two-legged posture and locomotion because these made possible the emergence of humanity's most vaunted distinctions, achievements, and problems. This seemingly purely physical rearrangement, in the opinion of anthropologists, made possible a new kind of life, human life, with all its new and improved features.

We are the only organisms that are both the creators and the beholders of beauty. We produce and find pleasure in music, dance, and all other forms of art and literature. We have created and continually re-create mathematics, science, medicine, philosophy, history, ethics, law, religion, industry, and our very civilization. These enormous achievements and sources of fulfillment, including our capacities for love, laughter, compassion, and self-awareness, to name a few, were suddenly made possible, perhaps even inevitable, when our hominid ancestors assumed the upright posture.[6]

The liberation of the forelimbs, no longer needed for support and locomotion, made possible the evolution of the human hand. The hand (*manus* in Latin) is a remarkable sensing instrument for assessing size, shape, texture, and weight. It is also a supremely versatile tool for *man*ufacturing, *man*ipulating, doing *man*ual labor, *man*aging, writing *man*uscripts, and even *man*dating. With our hands, we shape, create, caress, communicate, defend, hold, crush, and change the world around us in countless ways. In so doing, we often *man*acle ourselves in numerous figurative but *hand*icapping ways.

The mouth, no longer needed for grasping, carrying, or combat, became available for conversion into part of the speech apparatus.[7] These innovations provoked, facilitated, and accompanied the enormous development of the brain, without which the innovations would have been valueless for want of interpretation of sensory input and planning of motor output.

Together, these innovations made possible an immense repertoire of unprecedented capabilities that have produced and continue to produce diverse and ever-evolving cultures and civilizations. With our remarkable capacities for observation, reason, learning, and wonder (the last of which, according to Goethe, is the highest that humans can attain);[8] with our abilities to explore, modify, and adapt to diverse environments; and with our capability to communicate, to imagine, to invent, and to create, we have been able to inhabit the entire surface of the earth—mountaintops and valleys, vast continents and tiny islands, tropical rain forests and Arctic glaciers, deserts and rocky coasts—and may someday colonize other planets and interplanetary space. Contrast this with most other species that remain in the circumscribed areas to which they became adapted over the many millennia, at least until they are driven out by human exploitation of their habitats.

ENVIRONMENTS: NATURAL AND MAN-MADE

What is more, through the human ability to change our physical, sociocultural, and technological environments and to travel rapidly from one environment to another, we continually challenge and often exceed our adaptive capacities, presenting ourselves with health problems not encountered in other species.[9]

The rapid succession of self-challenges and changing environments that confront us with problems of adaptation is easily dramatized by noting the changes in the ways of life that have occurred in a single lifetime—mine, for example. The contrast between the high-tech, motorized, electronic, space-age, computerized, nuclear, jet-propelled world in which we live today and the one of my early childhood is impressive. In my South Philadelphia neighborhood, telephones, radios, refrigerators (other than iceboxes), and even electric lighting in the home were virtually unknown. At that time, television was only a fantasy in some would-be inventor's mind. A passing auto was still a cause for excitement and the taunt, "Get a horse!" (Despite the taunts, it was still a privilege to be invited for a ride in a neighbor's "Tin Lizzie.") I can also remember that people came charging out of their homes and workplaces just to watch the miracle of a plane (sometimes trailing a Lucky Strike banner) passing overhead.

As a student in junior high school, I built for my family and some of our neighbors their first radios (crystal sets) by winding my own variometer and variocoupler coils on toilet paper tubes and Quaker Oats cartons. I graduated to tube sets when the first triode vacuum tubes became available. I remember stealing off to the freight station to watch the telegrapher at work in wonder and to hear the click-clack of the telegraph and sending-key speaking in Morse code.

Thanks to human inventiveness, such changes in the ways of life occur much more rapidly than adaptive evolutionary changes can take place in our biological mechanisms. The challenge to human intelligence is to make adaptive behavioral changes that will protect those mechanisms and minimize potential damage.

I encountered many astonishing examples of the relentless tug-of-war between bold, adventurous human inventiveness and conservative, recalcitrant human biology during World War II. As a senior physiologist under the auspices of the Office of Scientific Research and Development and the US War Department, I was engaged in medical research related to the military. The basic and quite pervasive problem I was there to solve was that the machines of war were often designed and constructed with too little regard for the humans who were to operate them. For example, the first project in aviation medicine presented to our research team was to raise the human "ceiling" to match that of the aircraft. One of the most advanced pursuit planes of the time, the Thunderbolt, also known as a P-47, could fly above fifty thousand feet. At that altitude, the atmospheric pressure is so low (cabins were not pressurized in those days) that even 100 percent oxygen delivered by face mask could not load the blood with sufficient oxygen to sustain consciousness or even life. In addition, survival from a bailout at those altitudes was highly improbable, if not impossible.

Other examples of the disparity between man and machine were encountered during my research with the Signal Corps. The hand generators that provided electrical power for the radio transceivers on the battlefield required so much muscular power that only a corps of Arnold Schwarzeneggers could operate them for more than a few minutes at a time. What is more, the sound generated by the gears was almost perfect for binaural (two-ear) localization. As a result, operators were easy targets for enemy snipers. Similarly, early radar scopes were apparently designed with a total disregard or ignorance of the anatomy of the human neck and the functional properties of the human eye; there were disastrous consequences to the well-being of the operators and, hence, to the value of the radar system itself.

QUADRUPED TO BIPED, OR CONVERTING A CANTILEVER BRIDGE TO A SKYSCRAPER

The assumption of the erect stance and bipedal (two-legged) locomotion by our hominid ancestors was certainly a crucial step in the evolution of our greatest distinction from all other animals—human intelligence and all that it enables us to do. As stated previously in this chapter, the liberation of the forelimbs and mouth favored a great leap in brain development and made it possible for us to utilize our hands effectively and to develop speech and communication. This, in turn, opened the way for the evolution of culture and civilization as well as their attendant problems.[10]

Now, I want you to seriously consider how the upright posture has directly affected intrinsic human biology. Is a health-related price being paid for this seemingly simple rearrangement of bodily framework? Forget for a moment the technological and environmental unintended by-products previously discussed in this chapter as you consider this question.

Well, consider this. If we convert the billion-plus years that living forms have been evolving on planet Earth to a twenty-four-hour day, then humans came on the scene within the last few minutes. During that time, they stood up on their hind legs. That seems as daring a step as that of the first fish coming out of the water onto land. In taking that step, our predecessors were abandoning quadruped (four-legged) posture and locomotion despite its having been the very successful product of hundreds of millions of years of evolution. The quadruped frame has been described as an arched cantilever bridge (the spine) sturdily supported on a broad base provided by four pillars. The low center of gravity further enhances spinal stability. The pelvis of the quadruped is a freely moving rear end that supports no weight, and the head is suspended out front by strong muscles and thick ligaments.[11] The internal organs hang from the supple arched cantilever, very much like laundry on a clothesline flapping freely in the wind.

In a mere moment of evolutionary time, the early hominids started to convert this magnificent cantilever bridge to a skyscraper while retaining essentially the same component parts.[12] Despite altered forms and interrelationships, the human's component parts can be matched with those of other animals, bone for bone, joint for joint, ligament for ligament, tendon for tendon, and artery for artery, as undergraduate biology students discover in comparative anatomy. In other words, as Charles Darwin stated in *The Descent of Man*, "Man still bears in his bodily frame the indelible stamp of his lowly origin."[13]

(Given the sexist idiom of his day, we can assume that Darwin implied that woman bears the same stamp.) From an engineering viewpoint, it is axiomatic, and if it isn't it, should be: If you are going to build a sky-scraper, you should use skyscraper parts and not bridge parts.

THE MUSCULOSKELETAL PROBLEMS IN BEING VERTICAL

The former bridge is now a tall vertical structure with a high center of gravity balanced on a narrow base. The formerly cantilevered arch is now a vertical column subject to compressive, shearing, and twisting forces. The pelvis has become a major weight-bearing device, sup-porting everything above it.

The sacrum at the back of the pelvis and formerly merely the hind end of a wiggly horizontal spinal column is now its base. It supports the spinal column and everything that the pelvis supports, while being precariously suspended between the two ilia (hip bones). Is there any wonder that sacroiliac problems are so common among humans?

The large lumbar vertebrae in humans are markedly wedged in shape, thus creating *lumbar lordosis*, or the forward arching of the lower back; each vertebra tends to slide off the one below with the bottom one, the fifth lumbar vertebra, tending to slip off the top of the sacrum. The muscles of the back are called on not only for motion but also for the stabilization of the spine. Hence, the prevalence of low back pain among humans.

The muscular and ligamentous strain of keeping the segmented column from toppling and the lumbar vertebrae from slipping is responsible for much of the back pain that is our most prevalent com-plaint. Hips, knees, and feet are also extremely vulnerable, bearing as they do most or all of our body weight. Pain in these parts is also too familiar. In our studies on hundreds of apparently healthy medical stu-dents over a twenty-year period, we never encountered a student in whom we did not find objective evidence of invertebral or other mus-culoskeletal dysfunction.[14]

THE VISCERAL PROBLEMS IN BEING VERTICAL

I have another question I would like you to consider: Are there any consequences to circulation and other functions of the internal organs from assuming an upright stance? As was stated about the four-legged animals, the abdominal and pelvic viscera hang freely from the vertebral column. In two-legged man, these viscera tend to pile into the pelvic bowl, one upon the other. Drainage vessels, such as the veins and lymphatic vessels, may be compressed by the weight of the organs, contributing to congestion, stasis, edema (accumulation of fluid in the tissues), and their effects on visceral function. Hemorrhoids, another consequence of the damming of blood flow in the veins, are also a unique and common problem for humans. Other gravitational effects are the predisposition to hernia, and prolapse and retroversion of the uterus.

As for the circulation of the blood, the major blood vessel circuits in the quadruped are mainly in the horizontal plane. In the upright human, these circuits are largely vertical. Arterial blood needs to be pumped upward, against gravity, to the head and its contents. Tall columns of venous blood must be lifted from the feet through long veins in the legs and trunk back to the heart. Given time and with the addition of prolonged standing, inactivity, and poor muscular tone, the very weight of these columns distends the veins in the legs and often causes their valves to leak, resulting in painful varicosities that are yet another problem unique to man and related to the vertical stance.

However, we are not always vertical. Approximately one-third of our lives are spent in the horizontal position, and that presents still another circulatory problem. Visualize a man who has been recumbent for seven or eight hours suddenly called upon to spring to his feet and prepare for action (whatever that action might be). If the complex reflex adjustments to this sudden shift back to skyscraper status are at all sluggish, the brain, which is effectively housed in the penthouse, is deprived of blood, and the well-known consequences of fainting may result. Also problematic is that brain circulation in the upright person must be maintained without benefit of valves in the large veins of the head to arrest the downward rush of blood.

The respiratory system is also affected by verticality. Because of the downward angle of the ribs, drawing air into the lungs requires more muscular effort in the human than in quadrupeds since the ribcage must be lifted with each inspiration. Drainage of secretions in the bronchial tree is also upward and against the downward pull of gravity; hence, humans have an increased dependence on upward sweeping by the cilia (microscopic whiplike structures in the lining of the respiratory tubing), on the muscular action of the tiny bronchioles, and by coughing. Every lecturer, actor, concert artist, and symphony conductor is unavoidably aware of the intrusive din of coughing in audiences. How often is the interval between the first and second movements of a symphony prolonged while the conductor waits for the explosion of pent-up coughs to subside?

A similar challenge is presented to the sinuses on either side of the nose. The position of the sinus openings is such that in the upright position drainage by gravity is virtually impossible; each sinus requires a different orientation of the head to effect drainage. The uniquely human prevalence of sinusitis attests to the fact that this problem, too, remains to be solved by human ingenuity or by further evolution.

THE HELPLESSNESS OF THE HUMAN INFANT

Finally, the threat of an obstetrical impasse presented by the upright stance might have resulted in the extinction of the human species had it not been resolved by the evolutionary process. It also had an enormous impact on subsequent human evolution. The conversion of the pelvis into a major weight-bearing part of the skeleton necessitated its structural reinforcement. This was accomplished by a gradual thickening and a reduced flare of the pelvic bones. Unfortunately, this change began to encroach on the birth canal. Further, this adjustment transpired at a time when the gradual enlargement of the infant head, thanks to the blossoming cerebral cortex, required an even more spacious birth canal.

How did Mother Nature solve this problem? By advancing parturition (delivery) to such an immature stage of fetal development that the head could more easily pass through the narrowed canal. Thus, while the brain of the newborn baboon, for example, is almost as large as it is going to be (three-fourths of the adult weight), that of the human infant is only one-fourth of its ultimate, adult weight. The result of this change is that most of human brain development occurs after birth. Therefore, the human child is utterly helpless and dependent for a long time in contrast to the young ape, which can soon fend for itself.

Since most of the development of the human brain occurs outside the relatively constant environment of the uterus, each brain's postnatal development is profoundly influenced by all the environments, circumstances, events, people, teachings, ideas, beliefs, and cultural influences encountered as the youngster and his or her brain mature. These numerous and highly variable external factors influence the elaboration of the brain's circuitry. By circuitry, I mean the interconnections among the tens of billions of brain cells and the functional coalitions that they form. The child's brain, and therefore the mind, has a high degree of plasticity, as neuroscientists have observed. That is, it is subject to wiring and rewiring. Indeed, the development of these innumerable synaptic interconnections, together with the enlargement of the brain cells themselves, accounts for most of the postnatal increase in brain size.

Since the constellations of impinging influences are unique for each maturing person, they contribute enormously, along with heredity, to the uniqueness of the individual and the diversity of humankind. These influences serve, with varying degrees of success and with diverse results, to prepare the person for life as a social being and for his or her role in society, whether it be one born into or moved into. These postnatal influences also determine whether, and with what degree of competence, the person assumes responsibility for his or her own health.

DID WE GET A BAD DEAL?

These few examples of biomechanical problems associated with bipedal locomotion are also part of the cost of the great benefits to and the achievements of the human species. Other costs have been previously illustrated. Therefore, the issue is not that we got a bad deal and pay too high a price for the advantages of being human. The fact is that we had no choice in what evolution handed us.

However, we do have a choice in what we do with it and even, as some have declared, in the course of our future evolution. The real issue is this: Given human intelligence, creativity, problem-solving ability, ingenuity, resourcefulness, and so on, what can we do, individually and collectively, to lower the cost and increase the benefits of being human? Beginning with our children, what can be done through education, for example, to bring about less costly and more healthful and rewarding personal behavior? What can be done to our total physical and sociocultural environment to favor a more healthful societal behavior? Perhaps there are some lessons to be learned from individuals and cultures that have been relatively successful in this regard. These and related questions will be addressed in succeeding chapters.

At this point, though, and just for fun, I would like to conclude this discussion with a bit of doggerel that I wrote in 1948 when I was beginning to understand the relation of the human framework to human health. At that time, there was a rapid increase in the diseases we get, while the major medical focus was on the diseases we catch.

Psycho and Somatics

or

What Is Somata with the Psyche?

'Pon hind legs man's learned to stand,
Setting free his tongue and hand,
Favoring growth of seething brain,
Courting curse of spinal strain.

Maladapted to vertical stance,
Body lagging behind brain's advance,
Man shoots his bolts at microbial marauders—
And lives to die from degenerative disorders.

INHERITED EMOTIONS AND BEHAVIORS: OLD RESPONSES TO NEW ENVIRONMENTS

The problem of adaptation to our own creations is further complicated by the fact that we have inherited not only a biological apparatus seen in our cells, tissues, organs, and metabolic processes, but also emotional and behavioral patterns as well as their accompanying physiological changes. Indeed, it is helpful to think of emotions as triggering complex patterns of physiological responses that prepare us for action appropriate to the situation.[15] Like the protective and life-preserving mechanisms that we share with other forms of animal life, these behavioral mechanisms are also the products of millions of years of evolution. They have survived and been inherited by us because, like the other mechanisms, they had critical survival value under the conditions in which they evolved. The problem is that they are often inappropriate in the very different circumstances of human life today.

For example, anger and fright triggered in the wild by the sight or scent of a predator or adversary in turn triggers physiological preparations for "fight or flight," a perfectly appropriate and often life-saving response to a real life-threatening situation in the seas or the wilderness. However, we use the same behavioral mechanisms in human life in our cities, offices, factories, automobiles, airplanes, temperature-controlled homes, cocktail parties, classrooms, conference halls, meeting rooms, libraries, restaurants, theaters, ballparks, and beds, where the threat to life and to physical integrity is rare. Our ingrained response in these circumstances is not to objective reality (whatever that is), but to our perceptions.[16]

What is the adaptive value when the threat is not physical but perceptual, symbolic, verbal, social, or imagined? What about when the threat, real or imagined, is not to life and limb but to self-esteem, dignity, social standing, prestige, livelihood, or respect of one's children? When the fear is not of bodily damage but of failure—in the next examination, in business, in bed, on the golf course, or in the stock market? When the threat, real or not, is not in the immediate vicinity but in the boss's office thirty stories up, at home ten miles from the office, or in Washington, Moscow, the Persian Gulf, or Wall Street? What if the anger is provoked not by physical attack but by a word, slogan, epithet, discourtesy, insult, snub, reprimand, withdrawal of a privilege, or any real or fantasized injustice?

What does the physiological preparation for violence or flight accomplish in these situations? In what way, if any, do increased pumping action of the heart, increased blood pressure, diversion of the blood from the internal organs to the muscles, tightening of the muscles, sweating of the palms, drying of the mouth, accelerated blood clotting, dilation of the pupils, and secretion of adrenalin and other stress hormones enable us to make an adaptive response to any of the above situations? Physical combat and flight have been ruled out by civilized convention, except in war and sport. Thus, these physiological preparations for violence and exertion serve little if any adaptive purpose. They are not only useless but harmful responses; the biological engine races, while the vehicle remains at the curb. Under these circumstances, the only possible use of these physiological preparations would be to "blow off steam" unnecessarily generated in the first place.[17]

Hence, ancient biological defense mechanisms may in human life be turned against the person (very much like an autoimmune disease, such as rheumatoid arthritis, in which one's own tissues are fought off and destroyed), so may our behavioral mechanisms be destructive of self. Living in anger or fear can be enormously corrosive to health, well-being, and life itself.[18] The challenge to human intelligence is to learn to use these deeply ingrained patterns in ways that are adaptive to the situation. That is, we should develop behavior patterns that are appropriate to the current challenges of human life and that support health, well-being, and longevity.[19] The same is true of other patterns of thinking, feeling, and behaving inherited in the course of our individual development that we may employ inappropriately with detriment to our health.

STRESS

The concept of stress introduced by endocrinologist Hans Selye in the 1940s is closely related to the human behavioral misuse and abuse of response patterns inherited from our evolutionary predecessors.[20] Selye developed his ideas on stress from studies on rats and other lower mammals. (I shall use *stress* in this discussion as it is used colloquially. The correct word in this context, according to Selye's terminology, would be stressors, which are the external stimuli or demands; he defined *stress* as the response to the stressor.)

Since it was first introduced, stress has became such a popular idea that the public has been inundated with books, magazine articles, programs, courses, workshops, audiocassettes, videotapes, and pedantic platitudes about stress, stress management, and coping. We have somehow acquired the impression that stress is always harmful, despite Selye's emphasis on "stress without distress," and despite the fact that some of our favorite activities, including sports and sex, are happily stressful.

Stress has always been an intrinsic part of animal life. It is neither good nor bad; it is just an inevitable aspect of life. All animals, certainly all warm-blooded animals, are continually confronted with the natural and not always alarming stresses of finding food and water, dealing with adversaries and predators, finding mates, nourishing and protecting offspring, finding or contriving shelter, and surviving the extremes of weather. Stress may even be a part of the fun of play.

Modern society creates and confronts humans with a vastly larger and continually changing variety of stresses, such as those previously enumerated in my discussion of fear and anger. The biological impact of each stress, whether beneficial, harmful, or neutral, is determined not only by the nature and intensity of the external stimulus or demand (stressor) but by the personal meaning that we give it (principle IV). In other words, it is determined by our perception of it.[21] In turn, meaning and perception are influenced by all the values, biases, prejudices, habits, beliefs, feelings, and attitudes absorbed from our elders and our peers as we grow up and from the total culture in which we live and work. Of course, our own idiosyncrasies are also significant. We all wear colored glasses, and our outlook and the response to what we see are influenced by the tint of our cultural lenses.

STRESS OF THE PAST AND FUTURE

Unlike other animals, including advanced species of mammals, which as far as we can tell live only in the present, humans are often stressed by regrets, resentments, and guilt accumulated from the past and by worries about matters that have not yet, and perhaps never will, come to pass in the future. In short, all the circumstances in modern life that are stressful, usually meaning distressful, are stressful not in and of themselves but because we find them stressful or have made them stressful. Fortunately, our uniquely human intelligence enables us to change what we find by changing the color of our glasses and by creating personal and social worlds that enhance rather than erode health and well-being.

SUMMARY

1. Human health and illness are seen as products of evolution, with unique issues of adaptation to our modern environment, one both natural and man-made.

2. Human upright, two-legged posture and locomotion contribute unique challenges and advantages to human beings.

3. Inherited emotions and behaviors can be seen as old responses to new environments.

In the next chapter, we will explore the mixed blessings of human intelligence and its contribution to the origin of human vulnerability.

NOTES

1. E. J. Larson, *Evolution* (New York: Random House, 2004).

2. R. M. Nesse and G. C. Williams, *Why We Get Sick: The New Science of Darwinian Medicine* (New York: Vintage, 1994).

3. L. H. Caporale, *Darwin in the Genome: Molecular Strategies in Biological Evolution* (New York: McGraw-Hill, 2003).

4. M. Ridley, *Nature via Nurture: Genes, Experience, and What Makes Us Human* (New York: HarperCollins, 2003).

5. S. Jones, *Darwin's Ghost: The Origin of Species Updated* (New York: Ballantine, 2000).

6. W. H. Calvin, *A Brief History of the Mind: From Apes to Intellect and Beyond* (New York: Oxford University Press, 2004), pp. 15–22.

7. Ibid., pp. 83–106.

8. J. W. Goethe and J. P. Eckermann, *Conversations of Goethe with Johann Peter Eckermann*, trans. J. Oxenford and ed. J. K. Moorhead (New York: Da Capo, 1998).

9. J. M. Schwartz and S. Begley, *The Mind and the Brain: Neuroplasticity and the Power of Mental Force* (New York: HarperCollins, 2002), pp. 365–76.

10. J. C. Eccles, *Evolution of the Brain: Creation of the Self* (New York: Routledge, 1989), pp. 39–70; R. Leakey, *The Origin of Humankind* (New York: Basic Books, 1994).

11. H. F. Farfan, "The Biomechanical Advantage of Lordosis and Hip Extension for Upright Activity. Man as Compared with Other Anthropoids," *Spine* 3 (1978): 336–42.

12. G. Noone and W. T. Ang, "The Inferior Boundary Condition of a

Continuous Cantilever Beam Model of the Human Spine," *Australasian Physical & Engineering Sciences in Medicine* 19 (1996): 26–30.

13. C. Darwin, J. Moore, and A. Desmond, *The Descent of Man* (New York: Penguin Classics, 2004).

14. B. Peterson, ed., *The Collected Papers of Irvin M. Korr* (Colorado Springs, CO: American Academy of Osteopathy, 1979).

15. E. M. Sternberg, *The Balance Within: The Science Connecting Health and Emotions* (New York: W. H. Freeman, 2000), pp. 206–10.

16. H. Selye, *The Stress of Life* (New York: McGraw-Hill, 1976).

17. C. Charnetski and F. X. Brennan, *Feeling Good Is Good for You* (New York: St. Martin's, 2001), pp. 69–78.

18. D. Colbert, *Deadly Emotions: Understand the Mind-Body-Spirit Connection That Can Heal or Destroy You* (Nashville: Nelson Books, 2003).

19. S. I. Greenspan and S. G. Shanker, *The First Idea: How Symbols, Language, and Intelligence Evolved from Our Primate Ancestors to Modern Humans* (Cambridge, MA: Da Capo Press, 2004), pp. 253–56.

20. H. Selye, "Stress and Disease," *Science* 122 (1955): 625–31.

21. T. Bennett-Goleman, *Emotional Alchemy: How the Mind Can Heal the Heart* (New York: Harmony Books, 2001), p. 315.

Chapter 9

OTHER MIXED BLESSINGS OF HUMAN INTELLIGENCE

"The more nearly that time runs out, the less hurried I am."
—I. M. Korr

In this chapter, I'd like you to consider what mixed blessings human inventiveness has brought us. The natural answer is, of course, many mixed blessings occur in several categories and are probably familiar to most readers. Indeed, much has been written and said about them in recent years, especially in relation to preventing heart disease, cancer, stroke, and other afflictions.[1] Very little more, therefore, needs to be said about our mixed blessings here, except to place them in the context of this chapter's theme and in relation to the promotion of health and healthy old age. As we have seen thus far, the promotion of health transcends and incorporates the prevention of disease.

NUTRITION

Animals in the wild, whether they be herbivores, carnivores, insectivores, or omnivores (respectively, eaters of plants, flesh of other animals, insects, or combinations thereof), survive and thrive on the foods that they find in their habitat and that they consume in their natural state. Omnivorous humans, on the other hand, may in the same meal sample food from a Colorado mountain stream; the depths of the Pacific or Indian Ocean; produce farms in Iowa, Nebraska, New Jersey, and Pennsylvania; a ranch in Argentina; a dairy farm in Wisconsin; a forest floor in France; vineyards in California; orchards in New Zealand and Hawaii; and olive groves in Greece. Furthermore, most of the food has been prepared, cooked, seasoned, mixed, and altered in ways that not only satisfy nutritional requirements but also esthetic, ethnic, religious, fashionable, or other social, cultural, and economic considerations. It is extremely unlikely that the gastrointestinal system has ever been challenged to digest such a variety of foods in such combinations and concoctions, or in such quantities, in the entire course of our evolution.[2] Is there any reason to wonder that our digestive systems (among others) have cause to rebel so often?

As though that were not enough, we introduce into our foods and thence into our tissues synthetic or other substances, like the so-called additives, that do not naturally occur in our foods or in our bodies. These substances are introduced into our food at various stages during or after being grown, harvested, prepared, packaged, or displayed.[3] The purposes of these added substances are manifold: they are used to increase yield, reduce a producer's cost and effort, prolong shelf life, improve appearance, enhance flavor, accelerate growth, fatten livestock, increase salability, and swell profits.

Additives include, among others, various preservatives, herbicides, pesticides, insecticides, antibiotics, hormones, fertilizers artificial flavoring, coloring, sweeteners, and salt and other minerals. Some are known to be carcinogenic or hazardous to our health in other ways, especially when repeatedly consumed over long periods of time. The effects of some on our bodies and our overall health have yet to be determined.[4]

Conversely, we often remove essential nutrients from our foods, calling it refining, then restore them, calling the food enriched. Guided too often by taste, cost, convenience, or other nonnutritional considerations, we live on diets that are grossly unbalanced, excessive in empty calories, and lacking in essential components. To regain those lost essential components, we seek to replace them with costly and usually ineffectual or even harmful supplements.[5]

OTHER SUBSTANCES INHALED AND INGESTED

Humans are the only known organisms that deliberately take into their bodies, often in large daily quantities, substances that they know to be harmful, poisonous, and causative of disabling disease and premature death. In addition, we consume other disease-causing substances that induce behavior that is often disabling, that is threatening to life and limb of self and others, and that alienates one from fellow members of the species.

So why is it that we as humans adopt such practices? The answer is quite simple—because their effects feel good, momentarily. In other words, these substances induce pleasant changes in our mood and are the result of social custom and personal habit. I refer, of course, to tobacco and alcohol. Let me make it clear that I intend no moral judgment on those who use these substances. After all, although I am no longer a smoker, I did smoke for more than thirty years, and I will openly admit that I enjoy almost daily a glass of wine, beer, or highball. My concern is for the cost in human life, health, and well-being and for the enormous burden of disease and misery caused by the abusive use of these substances.[6]

According to former surgeon general C. Everett Koop, cigarette smoking is "the chief, single avoidable cause of death in our society, and the most important health issue of our time."[7] It is greater, even, than the spreading epidemic of AIDS. As for alcohol, the consequences related to its consumption, such as human illness and premature death; disabilities, disfigurements, and deaths occurring on our highways; and family dysfunction and social illness, are also well known and need no elaboration from me.

The same things can be said for heroin, cocaine, marijuana, and other addictive mind-altering drugs. I will add that the rampant abuse and misuse of medications in our culture must also be considered. This problem largely arises due to the unspoken consensus that every human complaint, illness, or disease can be chemically allayed or cured and that medicines are the sources of health. Forgotten also is that every desirable therapeutic or palliative effect of even our best medicines is part of a trade-off, with the price being undesirable side effects. Further, these effects may become dangerously exacerbated by the injudicious use of combinations of drugs by the same patient, a very common problem in the older population.[8]

My only purpose in the preceding paragraphs was not to belabor what is already widely known about chemical abuse but to illustrate once more that the most remarkable products of evolution—human intelligence as well as our capacities for observation, reason, invention, and experimentation—are too often employed with unintended consequences and a lack of critical evaluation. Have we reason to be scornful, even compassionately scornful, of the lemmings who are said to march off cliffs in droves to their deaths, of the occasional whale that swims into shallow water and dies flapping helplessly on some beach, or of the moth that incinerates itself in the candle flame? In what other ways can human intelligence be employed to help human beings "feel good," while contributing rather than robbing them of health?

STILL OTHER SUBSTANCES INHALED AND INGESTED

In addition to those toxic substances that we individually choose to take into our bodies, there are many others that we do not choose but that are imposed by our civilization. I have in mind:

1. The millions of tons of toxic chemicals discharged into our atmosphere by countless automobiles, trucks, airplanes, diesel

engines, fossil-fuel furnaces, incinerators, and industrial smokestacks. They are poisons absorbed with every breath.

2. The poisonous industrial wastes, garbage, sewage, heavy metals, and crude oil dumped into our seas, bays, lakes, rivers, and streams that pollute the water we drink and the food we take from those waters; these also contribute to the extinction of many species.

3. The radioactive and other hazardous wastes piled up in dumpsites that leak into the atmosphere, soil, and groundwater.

4. The volatile substances used as refrigerants and propellants in spray bottles that are finding their way into our upper atmosphere, where they are destroying the layers of ozone that shield us from overexposure to carcinogenic ultraviolet radiation.

5. The volatile poisons in building materials and furnishings in homes and workplaces.

6. The destruction of millions of acres of wilderness, wetlands, and rain forests. These areas are essential for the removal of accumulating carbon dioxide and the replenishment of oxygen as well as to the survival of thousands of animal species that inhabit them.

Are these and many other impediments to health and causes of disease the unavoidable side effects of civilization and technological advance? Are they the nonnegotiable price that must be paid for the advantages, wonders, pleasures, comforts, and conveniences of civilization? The answer is firmly in the negative. The same intelligence that gave us those cherished advances and advantages can also find ways to minimize the chemical and other hazards to public health. What is required is a public and governmental decision to accomplish precisely that and to give the effort the high priority it must have.

MUSCULOSKELETAL DISUSE

As was discussed in chapter 3 on structure function, the musculo-skeletal system is designed for action and for locomotion: swimming, leaping, dancing, lifting, carrying, pushing and pulling, creating beauty, making music, tilling, sowing and reaping, building and tearing down, and all the innumerable things that humans can do. In our automotive, automated, motorized, robotized, and computerized civilization, however, and in most occupations, the largest portion of this massive system has little demand and certainly little sustained demand placed upon it. For too many people, there is little muscular effort beyond pushing their brake and accelerator pedals, walking from one office to another, climbing a flight of stairs, lifting a child, fingering a keyboard, carrying an attaché case, throwing switches, or turning dials. We even have remote control devices to spare us the exertion of leaving our armchairs to change television channels. If we are tired at the end of the work day, few of us can claim muscular exertion as the cause.

The pathological consequences of inactivity have been studied extensively and were briefly summarized in the last section of chapter 3. Muscles atrophy, tighten, and weaken; joints stiffen; and bones lose density. With the loss of flexibility and muscular strength comes the loss of mobility. The diminished ease of motion discourages activity, which, in turn, favors further loss of mobility, and so forth, resulting in a downward spiral of musculoskeletal deterioration.[9] These changes are most evident in older people following retirement, but, as previously mentioned, experimental studies have shown that similar changes can occur in young people during prolonged inactivity. Indeed, the posture and shuffling gaits of these younger people, and even their moods, resemble those of much older persons.

Musculoskeletal inactivity also has serious consequences for the visceral systems. Dr. Walter M. Bortz and other distinguished gerontologists and geriatricians have shown that physical inactivity results in premature aging and deterioration as reflected in blood and body composition, in metabolism, and in nervous, cardiovascular, respiratory, digestive, and renal function.[10] Conversely, restoration of flexibility and mobility as well as resumption of physical activity results in rejuvenation even in very old people. Equally important is the widely experienced beneficial effect of physical activity on mental health and mood that has been documented in recent years by several large-scale, long-term studies.[11] Fortunately, unlike cigarette smoking and other addictions, addiction to inertia is readily subject to cure.

Certainly, my own continued good health and capacity for enjoyment in my eighties can, to a very large degree, be ascribed to almost daily vigorous physical activity. The increasing recognition of the contribution of regular exercise to complete physical, mental, and social well-being is evident in the growing number of people of all ages currently engaged in exercise programs, such as walking, jogging, swimming, and other aerobic exercise. It is evident too in the proliferation of health clubs and fitness centers as well as in the growth of the sporting goods industry. It is my opinion that the leadership of Dr. Kenneth H. Cooper and other specialists in exercise physiology and sports medicine should be gratefully acknowledged for the aerobic exercise movement.[12]

In summary, human technological advances can have global unintended consequences, including problems with human nutrition, substance abuse, and musculoskeletal disuse, which can be viewed as the other mixed blessings of human intelligence.

In this section, we have discussed the origins of human vulnerability and challenged your thoughts and beliefs regarding your interface with your environment, including that with your healthcare system, and the machinery that you "inherited." It is now time for us to begin to lay out a strategy in part 4 to employ our uniquely human capabilities to create health and well-being so that I can share the natural joy that I have come to experience in living long and loving it.

NOTES

1. T. H. Holmes and R. H. Rahe, "The Social Readjustment Rating Scale," *Journal of Psychosomatic Research* 11 (1967): 213–18; R. M. Sapolsky, *Why Zebras Don't Get Ulcers* (New York: W. H. Freeman, 1998); H. Selye, *The Stress of Life* (New York: McGraw-Hill, 1976); A. Toffler, *Future Shock* (New York: Bantam, 1971); A. Weil, *Spontaneous Healing* (New York: Ballantine, 1995), pp. 154–70; H. Benson and M. Z. Klipper, *The Relaxation Response* (New York: Avon, 1976).

2. A. S. Truswell, "ABC of Nutrition: Some Principles," *British Medical Journal*, clinical research ed. 291 (1985): 1486–90.

3. A. Furst, "Can Nutrition Affect Chemical Toxicity?" *International Journal of Toxicology* 21 (2002): 419–24.

4. T. Sugimura, "Nutrition and Dietary Carcinogens," *Carcinogenesis* 21 (2000): 387–95.

5. A. Weil, *Healthy Aging: A Lifelong Guide to Your Physical and Spiritual Well-Being* (New York: Knopf, 2005), pp. 141–76.

6. E. Single et al., *International Guidelines for Estimating the Costs of Substance Abuse* (Ontario: Canadian Centre on Substance Abuse, 1996).

7. C. E. Koop, "The Health Consequences of Nicotine Addiction: A Report of the Surgeon General," US Department of Health and Human Services 1988, http://www.cdc.gov/tobacco/sgr/sgr_1988/index.htm (accessed March 1, 2007).

8. W. R. Hazzard et al., *Principles of Geriatric Medicine and Gerontology*, 4th ed. (New York: McGraw-Hill, 2000), p. 326.

9. H. Sandler, *Inactivity: Physiological Effects*, ed. J. Vernikos (New York: Academic Press, 1986).

10. W. M. Bortz II, "Disuse and Aging," *Journal of the American Medical Association* 248 (1982): 1203–208.

11. National Institute on Aging, "Baltimore Longitudinal Study of Aging," June 10, 2005, http://www.grc.nia.nih.gov/branches/blsa/blsa.htm (accessed March 1, 2007); J. L. Fleg et al., "Accelerated Longitudinal Decline of Aerobic Capacity in Healthy Older Adults," *Circulation* 112 (2005): 674–82; A. J. Vita et al., "Aging, Health Risks, and Cumulative Disability," *New England Journal of Medicine* 338 (1998): 1035–41.

12. K. Cooper, *Running without Fear* (New York: M. Evans, 1985).

PART 4

CREATING YOUR WELL-BEING

"The more I remain me, the more I change; the more I change, the more I become me."

—I. M. Korr

Chapter 10
COMMITMENT, DISCIPLINE, MOTIVATION

"The more I choose to be bound by the laws of nature, the freer I become."

—I. M. Korr

Given human intelligence, imagination, creativity, reason, resourcefulness, ingenuity, ability to define and solve problems, and so on, what can we do, individually and collectively, to lower the cost and increase the benefits of being human? The premise underlying this question is that the kinds of minds that have created our technological civilization can solve the problems and the side effects generated by that civilization. By side effects, I mean the negative impact on health and quality of life as well as the threats to the survival of the human race and other species. Surely human minds can guide us from behavior that is self-defeating, even suicidal and lemminglike, to behavior that is more likely to continue the cultural evolution begun in the Paleolithic era some forty thousand or fifty thousand years ago and, hence, fulfill the human potential.

It seems to me that any strategy for the improvement of individual, family, community, and world health must have its foundation not only in (1) the biological components, processes, and mechanisms that humans share with other creatures, but also in (2) the distinctively human contexts in which the components function, (3) the physical and sociocultural environments in which humans function, and (4) the uniqueness of each individual.

The opportunity as well as the responsibility to strike a better balance between costs and benefits on behalf of human health is shared by individuals, communities, institutions, governments, and international bodies. However, as has been said again and again in the foregoing pages, the primary responsibility for health lies with the individual possessor guardian of the intrinsic biological resources on which health, its maintenance, recovery, and improvement depend. After all, these personal indwelling resources constitute the fundamental healthcare system on which all others rely and without which they are all powerless. The responsibilities of society and its agencies are (1) to prepare and enable individuals to assume *their* responsibility and (2) to create, guard, and maintain the environments that will allow our personal healthcare systems to operate at their very best.

Therefore, in part 4 I intend to address the opportunity each person has to move to a physiological path that leads to healthier, more fulfilling, and longer life. For this purpose, I again draw on the lessons learned from my own experiences and those of other healthy, active old people. In offering these guides to the reader, I do not assert that they are the only, the best, or the most reliable means, only that they have worked for me and for other men and women who have enjoyed long, healthy, productive, fulfilling lives.

I hasten to emphasize that what follows is not merely a set of directions on how to get healthy. Many "how-to-do-its" are already available, each focusing on one or another "it," such as diet, exercise, stress management, and so on. The purpose of this book remains to offer knowledge about human biology and behavior as well as the principles that underlie all of the effective measures. In this way, I mean to help each person, in his or her own way, to find more healthful ways of thinking, behaving, being, and becoming.

I believe that each person seeking better health must discover what specifically works best for herself or himself. I seek to offer guidelines for such discoveries. The question in each reader's mind should be "What way of life will enable me to more fully express my individuality, to enjoy life, and to achieve my highest potential?" There is, however, one indispensable element without which the quest for what works would be only perfunctorily (and unrewardingly) pursued, if at all. It is the subject of the next segment of this chapter.

COMMITMENT TO ONE'S HEALTH

The most essential element, but not necessarily the first in sequence, is a total commitment to one's own health. I do not recall that I ever consciously declared my commitment before starting on what eventually became my chosen path. I am aware only that I became committed soon after embarking on the path.

That time also marked the beginning of what I have described in the first chapter as my transformation. I know that the impetus for my commitment to the improvement of my health came soon after my first few steps on the new path when I discovered how good it felt. Little did I know how good it was going to feel or for how long.

It has been my experience that people are turned on when they find themselves moving through a barrier or a limitation that they had resignedly accepted as permanent and as the inevitable result of some unfortunate circumstance of heredity or of advancing age.

Commitment is essential to healthy living because it generates another essential element, the subject of the next segment.

SELF-DISCIPLINE

When I discovered that I could convert the principles that underlie the practice of osteopathic medicine into a guide for healthy living, I chose to adopt them as a way of life, a disciplined way of life. For me, this meant controlled, goal-directed behavior, with my goal being the enhanced quality of life that accompanies high-level health.

I tried with audiences of older people many years later to stress the importance of self-discipline in healthy living, but I encountered immediate resistance. Self-discipline, it seems, has negative connotations of self-denial and enforced obedience to a forbidding list of *thou-shalt-nots*. I eventually learned not to press this point. However, despite what people think and without being identified as such, self-discipline follows quite naturally once commitment is made.

Not only is self-discipline *not* the constraining or relinquishing of pleasures, it is a liberating way of life. If a healthy discipline is employed, rather than an overly restrictive or unhealthy one, it becomes the structure from which one may find freedom within which to function. One lives, not in conflict, but in harmony with the natural, unremitting tendency of the bodymind toward what we call health. The energy thus saved becomes available for the enhancement and multiplication of pleasures rather than their denial. It is an interesting paradox that the more one chooses to be bound by nature's laws, the freer one becomes.

MOTIVATION

What motivates one to make such a commitment? Certainly, the mere wish for better health is not enough. In my experience, the most powerful motivators are the observable results and the good feelings that come soon after a trial run on the new path. For me, then in my forties, it was the vitality brought on by enhanced freedom of motion and ease of breathing.

More recently, I have learned that essentially the same motivators serve others, even or perhaps especially, older people who yearn for the mobility they once had and who find daily tasks becoming increasingly difficult because of the stiffness that is often mistakenly assumed to be arthritis. This discovery came several years ago in the guise of a friend who was then also in his mid-seventies. While I visited him in his home one evening, he confessed his envy of my mobility and vigor. He also wanted to know what he might do to improve his.

In response, I demonstrated a few of my routine flexibility exercises, which ended with me in the standing position and placing my palms on the floor while keeping my legs straight. To assess his flexibility, I then asked him to try to do the same thing and see how close he could come to touching his toes. As he left his chair, he laughed sardonically, saying, "I haven't been able to get below my knees for forty years!" In fact, because of the shortened muscles of his thighs, hips, and back, he was unable even to straighten his legs. Nevertheless, I asked him to hold the position so that the weight of his upper body could stretch the tight muscles. I also suggested that he "let go" a little with each exhalation and thereby deepen the stretch. Within a few minutes, his fingers began to migrate downward, almost reaching midshin. He straightened in amazement and asked how he could do the same for other parts of his body. Naturally, I proceeded to demonstrate.

As he later discovered, of course, the effect of that first effort was largely transient. However, encouraged by that evening's experience, he continued to do the simple exercises I taught him, with a resultant steady improvement in his mobility. As had been my experience many years earlier, the improved ease of motion induced him to resume physical activities that he had once enjoyed and to adopt other healthful changes in his lifestyle and behavior. Though in his late seventies, he too has enjoyed a transformation, and it allowed him to arrest and then reverse his downward trend on the health spectrum.

Months later, I asked him what had motivated him to make the commitment to improved health. After a moment's reflection, his response was that there were apparently three main factors. First, he said, was what he described as my example, one that had convinced him that his efforts could pay off, too. The second impetus was that he had in the toe-touching effort broken through a barrier that he had thought was fixed and permanent. Third, and this is the most important, he had done so by his own efforts, which had inspired a sense of confidence and of being in control. This, he said, had moved him to "take charge."

In more recent work with groups of elderly people, I have found the technique of demonstrating quick improvement in mobility by one's own efforts to be a powerful motivator as had been the case for my friend. I made it my practice to ask a member of each group which part of the body was most handicapped by stiffness; I then showed how to improve that area. Women seemed to be especially grateful for the restored mobility that enabled them to resume social, recreational, vocational, and volunteer activities. Housekeepers, for example, welcomed their renewed ability to reach upper shelves or to retrieve fallen objects that had rolled under a heavy item of furniture. One lady in her eighties jubilantly reported several weeks after beginning the recommended exercises that she had "discovered a treasure" of long-lost objects that had rolled under her bed.

Experiences such as mine (and those who have been encouraged by my example) have been reported in the literature by other researchers and by practitioners of sports medicine and rehabilitation. While attention to musculoskeletal flexibility may be less important for individuals who have been physically and vigorously active, I am convinced that restoration of mobility is vital for habitually sedentary persons, especially in older persons for whom exertion is difficult and unpleasant because of joint stiffness, muscular weakness, and cardiovascular and respiratory sluggishness.

In conclusion, I firmly believe that creating your own well-being involves commitment, self-discipline, and motivation (principle IV). While difficult to follow in theory, these traits naturally develop as one chooses to allow the process of change toward better health to occur. By observing active role models and breaking through the barriers of old beliefs, an inspired sense of confidence and of being in control can joyfully begin to take shape.

Chapter 11

FREEDOM OF MOTION

"The walls that surround us in our minds and within which we have been taught to live are as constraining as the tallest and strongest of stone walls. Yet they crumble and vanish when we walk through them."

—I. M. Korr

MY OWN EXPERIENCE

You may recall from chapter 1 that after I had discovered the pleasures of walking, running, cycling, and tennis, I asked Dr. Chace why he had never prescribed such exercises for me. His immediate answer was "In order for there to be motion, there must be freedom of motion. I knew that you would respond when you were ready."

How right he was! With my improvement in ease of motion, the impulse to move came spontaneously. It also brought with it a sense of achievement and self-confidence, both of which generated enormous pleasure. These new feelings apparently triggered my undeclared commitment to my health and the assumption of responsibility for my health. Through the succeeding years, I have maintained my ease of motion with periodic osteopathic manipulative treatments, which are now more like fine tuning and, in the past few years, with yoga exercises that I perform for about twenty minutes three times a week.

I do not intend to imply that improvement of bodily flexibility must precede an exercise program or that it is the only or the best motivator. My intention is simply to illustrate how it has served me well, and this includes others whom I have been able to influence.

MOBILITY AND ITS REWARDS

I would now like to convey some of the rich rewards of maintaining, restoring, and improving your bodily flexibility. The benefits of freedom of motion are not purely physical, solely limited to the body component of bodymind. As another expression of the oneness of the person or interactive unity, the benefits extend abundantly to the psychological, behavioral, and even visceral realms—hence, to the whole person. After all, the musculoskeletal system is more than a vehicle. It is or can be, among other things, an infinite source of pleasure and an instrument of self-expression.

As was my experience during my transformation, people who experience freedom of motion for the first time or who have recovered it, even late in life, are aware of a feeling of bounciness, of a spring in the step, of a sense of resiliency. These feelings are not purely subjective but also remarked upon by others. Somehow, by mechanisms we are just beginning to understand, this sense of buoyancy radiates to the mind and the spirit with powerful effects that favor lightness of mood, optimism, self-assurance, openness, and flexibility of mind.

As we all know, our bodily attitudes, as in our postures and the ways in which we move, communicate much about us and our mental attitudes. Further, they may reflect impressions we wish to convey to others and even aspects of ourselves that we wish to conceal or of which we are not aware. (I remember too well the posture—shoulders pulled back, chest thrust forward—that I had unconsciously adopted to convey to others a self-confidence I did not feel.) In time, the postures or bodily configurations we wear influence the impact that the relentless force of gravity has on our bodies. They determine the sites of strain and vulnerability, and it is no coincidence that the words *posture* and *attitude* apply to both the physical and the psychological realms.

MIND-MUSCLE INTERPLAY

Our changing mental and emotional tensions, both the pleasant and the unpleasant, are accompanied by corresponding patterns of muscular tension. Chronic tensions and unresolved emotional conflicts are reflected in sustained muscular contractions that may have deleterious consequences, such as pain, weakness, and fatigue. Those who emotionally feel "all knotted up" do, in fact, have knots in their bodies to prove it. The natural guarding response of our musculature to emotional trauma is fundamentally the same as that of the threat of physical trauma. The resistant or immobile component gets in the way of every motion called upon to participate; it is like the out-of-step marcher in a parade or the out-of-tune horn in the symphony.

The muscles and their neural controls are also a memory bank, an instrument for learning, for remembering, and for forgetting. All of the injunctions and thou-shalt-nots accumulated in our respective upbringings are recorded (*embedded* or *buried* may actually be more accurate) in our neuromuscular system as patterns of unconscious behavior and reflexive knee-jerk reactions. When these patterns are inappropriate in adult behavior or maladaptive to changing circumstances in our lives, as they too often are, they diminish our control of our behavior and responses, intrude in our interpersonal relationships, limit our options, and reduce our ability to acquire more appropriate patterns.

The development of musculoskeletal flexibility followed by the relaxation of chronic tensions and fixations facilitates the replacement of unsuitable behaviors with behaviors of our conscious choice. Often these musculoskeletal fixations are so deeply embedded and so self-sustaining that they may require highly skilled physical or psychotherapeutic intervention. Osteopathic physicians frequently have the experience, while manipulatively unraveling a knot in a patient's body, of releasing a cathartic emotional storm that manifests in a flood of tears, anger, or painful memories.[1] This phenomenon can be understood as a long-blocked healing process of bodymind being released. It has been described by Jack Painter, PhD, as a breach of the bodymind armor, inside which so many of us spend our lives.[2]

In a later chapter, I will describe the wonderful liberating effects of my body armor gradually eroding and falling off, revealing my knee-jerk, self-defeating behaviors that needed to be replaced.

RESEARCH FINDINGS

In chapter 2 in my discussion of interactive unity, or oneness of the person, I showed that the many parts of the body are in continuous and close communication with each other through the circulation of the blood and other body fluids and through the central nervous system. Each part influences and is influenced by the others. Nothing can go wrong with any part, certainly not a major part, without affecting the other parts and the person as a whole. Other parts most likely to be affected are (1) those that are sensitive to chemical agents released into the bloodstream by the dysfunctional organ or tissue and (2) those that receive their own nerve supply from the same levels of the spinal cord or brain stem.

This principle of interactive unity goes into effect when motion is impaired in a given joint or other musculoskeletal component, such as the fixations and muscular tensions discussed above. As the many years of research conducted by my colleagues and myself have shown, the patterns of sensory nerve impulses or feedback sent into the central nervous system by the affected joints, muscles, ligaments, and tendons are so exaggerated or garbled that an "irritable focus," described as a facilitated (hyperexcitable) segment, is established in that part of the central nervous system.[3] Since the central nervous system cannot organize an adaptive response to such unintelligible signals, what amounts to a holding pattern results, immobilizing that part of the body by sustained muscular contraction. This not only may be painful, as in backaches, but it also interferes with the coordination of motion and places burdens of compensation on other parts of the body. The consequences are especially serious when the immobilization is located in the weight-bearing parts of the musculoskeletal system, such as the spine or pelvis.

As though this were not enough, our research further showed that the distorted sensory input also influences the sympathetic nervous system. Sympathetic nerves that originate in the corresponding segments of the central nervous system are most affected. These sympathetic neurons (nerve cells), which have a powerful influence on blood flow and function, send nerve fibers to blood vessels throughout the body, including those in the central nervous system and all the internal organs.

Therefore, the blood vessels, organs, and tissues receiving their innervation (nerve supply) from the facilitated segments become targets of abnormal impulse patterns, with harmful effects. Among the most hazardous is constriction of blood vessels, including those in the brain and spinal cord, which results in ischemia (reduced blood flow) and hypoxia (insufficient oxygen). Of course, the clinical impact of this phenomenon depends on how long the abnormal impulses are permitted to continue as well as other circumstances in that person's life. Most important for my purposes, the impact of all unfavorable circumstances and emotional upsets will be magnified in tissues and organs subjected to the intensified bombardment. In a review study of the clinical literature, I showed that local or general sympathetic hyperactivity is a common factor in many diseases and ailments.[4]

Later research I conducted demonstrated that peripheral nerves, those supplying the tissues and organs of the body, not only deliver impulses and neurotransmitters to them but also supply trophic (nurturing) proteins manufactured in the nerve cells. These proteins are essential for normal tissue and organ function and even for the survival of some tissues. The synthesis of these proteins, their delivery, or both may be impaired by the kinds of musculoskeletal dysfunctions previously discussed, with harmful and sometimes irreversible effects on the neurologically related tissues and organs.[5] As devastating as this may sound, these effects can be prevented or remedied by the maintenance or restoration of mobility.

MOBILITY AND THE ENRICHMENT OF LIFE

Another total-person benefit that results from restoring and maintaining a high degree of mobility is that it enables us to continue our exposure to a variety of environments, sensory stimuli, and opportunities for learning. The benefit of access to a rich environment through mobility has been shown to favor the continued learning-related strengthening, rearrangement, and proliferation of synaptic connections among the brain cells.[6] Some of this research was reviewed in a recent "Mind and Body Special Issue" of *Time* magazine, titled "The Brain: A User's Guide."[7]

The flourishing of synaptic interconnections accounts for the relatively high capacity of the young to acquire new knowledge, understanding, and skills. This capacity declines with age, but only if we shield ourselves from new environments and new challenges by sedentary living. Given continued mobility, the "old dog" can be taught new tricks. Further, the capacity for continued creative and intellectual growth and development in old age has been richly documented in *The Fountain of Age* by Betty Friedan.[8]

At the age of sixty and indeed throughout my sixties, this old dog moved into what was, for me, a totally new field of research, experimental neurosurgery and radioactive isotope technology, which required the development of skills I did not have. However, the acquirement of these new skills enabled me and my colleagues to trace proteins synthesized in nerve cells as they moved down the length of the axons and, as we were the first to show, across the junctions into the muscle cells that they controlled. This research that disclosed a mechanism underlying the trophic functions of nerves was, I think, the best of my entire career.

At the age of sixty-six, I accepted the first of a long and continuing series of invitations to act as a consultant and lecturer in many parts of the world. In my late seventies, I began a most gratifying volunteer part-time career as a teacher of "eugeriatrics," my term for the art and science of healthy aging. (The response prompted the writing of this book, my first effort in writing for other than professional—scientific and medical—readers.)

In my eightieth winter, I took up cross-country skiing for the first time and have maintained and refined the newly acquired motor patterns as well as my fitness on the NordicTrack, an eightieth birthday gift. In the past year or so, I have been able to polish my freestyle stroke to the degree that I now swim with almost the same ease and pleasure that I have long enjoyed in walking.

In addition to learning new physical skills, service on the ethics committee of a large community hospital obliged me to undertake the serious study of bioethics in relation to the most difficult and controversial ethical issues of the day. Having retired from paid employment during the writing of this book, I have found other opportunities for challenging volunteer service, such as peer counseling and participation on boards and councils of local governmental and private agencies. These have required training and study in diverse and unfamiliar fields. My experiences very gratifyingly substantiate research that demonstrates that older subjects who regularly do aerobic exercise perform better on cognitive tests than do sedentary individuals of the same age with low aerobic fitness.[9]

The most adventurous and rewarding of my old-dog-learning-new-tricks experiences has been my remarriage at the age of seventy-six; it is a continuing adventure that has vastly enriched this, the best time, of my life.

In light of this last and personally gratifying example, it comes as no surprise to me that mobility also facilitates the maintenance and continued enrichment of social relationships. Extensive surveys of various human populations by Drs. House, Landis, and Umberson,[10] as well as experimental studies, have provided strong evidence for a close causal relationship between the quality and range of social relationships on the one hand and levels of health on the other. Social isolation is shown to be a major risk factor for mortality from many causes.

GAINING FREEDOM OF MOTION

Given these rich rewards, how does one go about improving flexibility? I am aware that many readers, even those who are already committed to health and are ready to take charge, may find the concepts of practice, exercises, and routines abhorrent. Certainly, most of us who were forced to take music lessons as children remember how boring the exercises were. We can recall as well what delight we felt when at last we heard ourselves playing real music. So it is for these exercises and this practice. The music of bodymind is even more heartwarming. With a slight adjustment of attitude, physical exercises can be fun, too, especially as one observes and enjoys the progressive improvement in flexibility, mobility, physical function, and overall health-related quality of life.

Those who resist setting a little time aside for exercises (even though the reward is a more fruitful and pleasant day) will find the sources listed below very helpful. The National Institute on Aging offers a comprehensive overview of not only flexibility exercises but also the benefits of endurance, balance, and strength training.[11] Guidelines on how to initiate a safe exercise program and suggestions for specific activities are outlined on this Web site. Bob Anderson's simply titled book *Stretching*[12] shows different stretching exercises, while, in my opinion, both young and old would enjoy following instructions in *Easy Does It Yoga* by Alice Christensen.[13] This charmingly illustrated little volume of yogic exercises includes sections on improvement of respiratory ease and efficiency and on relaxation techniques.

Before you begin any exercises, either those suggested in the resources listed above or those undertaken through your own initiative, it is important to take a moment to identify your immediate objective. Generally, that objective should be to increase, and in most cases this means restore, the range of motion of each joint. Specifically, I mean the shoulders, hips, and other joints of the extremities as well as and just as importantly those of the entire spinal column, meaning the joints between the vertebrae, and the pelvis. Ease of motion is increased by relaxing and lengthening the stiffened, shortened muscles that support and move these joints. This, in turn, is accomplished by stretching the muscles in every plane of motion. In hinge joints (the elbows and knees), we deal with one plane of motion and only flexor (bending) and extensor (straightening) muscles. In the joints (plural!) of the shoulder, however, we deal with a multiplicity of planes and muscles. The same is true of the intervertebral and pelvic joints. Hence, I hope that you can see the importance of following the guidance of those, such as the previously recommended authors, who have a sound knowledge of human anatomy and a thorough grounding in exercise techniques. You may also find it helpful to explore the many instructional programs offered by local YMCA and YWCA centers, senior centers, and fitness clubs.

In this chapter, we discussed freedom of motion and its importance for well-being. In the next chapter, we will discuss the much-maligned other biological factors of exercise, breathing, and diet and weight control.

NOTES

1. B. Nathan, *Touch and Emotion in Manual Therapy* (New York: Churchill Livingstone, 1999).

2. J. W. Painter, "Postural Integration, Transformation of the Whole Self," http://www.bodymindintegration.com/PItransformation.html (accessed March 16, 2007).

3. B. Peterson, ed., *The Collected Papers of Irvin M. Korr* (Colorado Springs, CO: American Academy of Osteopathy, 1979).

4. I. M. Korr, "Sustained Sympathicotonias as a Factor in Disease," in *The Neurobiologic Mechanisms in Manipulative Therapy*, ed. I. M. Korr (New York: Plenum, 1978), pp. 229–68.

5. Peterson, *Collected Papers*, pp. 91–118.

6. E. Goldberg, *The Wisdom Paradox: How Your Mind Can Grow Stronger as Your Brain Grows Older* (New York: Gotham, 2005); J. LeDoux, *Synaptic Self: How Our Brains Become Who We Are* (Middlesex, England: Penguin, 2002); J. M. Schwartz and S. Begley, *The Mind and the Brain: Neuroplasticity and the Power of Mental Force* (New York: Regan, 2002).

7. "Mind and Body Special Issue," *Time*, January 29, 2007.

8. B. Friedan, *The Fountain of Age* (New York: Simon and Schuster, 1993).

9. J. D. Churchill et al., "Exercise, Experience and the Aging Brain," *Neurobiology of Aging* 23 (2002): 941–55; C. Fabre et al., "Improvement of Cognitive Function by Mental and/or Individualized Aerobic Training in Healthy Elderly Subjects," *International Journal of Sports Medicine* 23 (2002): 415–21.

10. J. S. House, K. R. Landis, and D. Umberson, "Social Relationships and Health," *Science* 241 (1988): 540–45.

11. "National Institute on Aging," US National Institutes of Health, http://www.nia.nih.gov/ (accessed March 26, 2007).

12. B. Anderson, *Stretching* (Bolinas, CA: Shelter, 2000).

13. A. Christensen, *Easy Does It Yoga* (New York: Fireside, 1999).

Chapter 12

OTHER BIOLOGICAL FACTORS

"My body always strives to meet my expectations of it, good or bad."
—I. M. Korr

Before I turn to my discussion of three other fundamental biological factors that can be improved by our own efforts, I want to remind you that I specifically devoted an entire chapter to one of the biological factors, freedom of motion. My reasons are threefold. First, the enhancement of mobility has been, in my experience, a powerful motivator. Second, as I hope I have shown, ease of motion has a pervasive influence in that it facilitates the improvement of many other factors. Third, its importance to health and especially to healthy aging has been seriously underestimated and overlooked.

EXERCISE

Having discussed freedom of motion, the questions I would now like you to consider are (1) what kinds of motion and (2) how much? The importance of regular exercise to health has been so well established by research (these studies are so numerous and accessible that I will provide only a few references here)[1] and by experience, and so widely acknowledged by the general public (witness, for example, the proliferation of athletic clubs, fitness centers, and related industries) that there is no need for further justification. Further, in chapter 3 on the principle of structure and function, I showed that continuing musculoskeletal activity throughout life benefits not only that system but all the others as well. Since the muscles are the main consumers in the body economy, their use in physical activity throughout life places demands for service by the circulatory, respiratory, and other internal organ systems. These demands maintain both the muscles and the organ systems' functional capacities and generate a prosperous body economy. Putting the muscles to rest as we age not only diminishes our ease of motion,[2] but also hastens the decline of those internal organ systems and their ability to sustain life.[3]

In a review of recent gerontological research, T. Franklin Williams, MD, former director of the National Institute on Aging (one of the National Institutes of Health) and now a professor emeritus in the medical school at the University of Rochester, concluded, "When animal or human subjects who have maintained a good level of exercise into later years are compared with younger animals or humans, functional declines previously attributed to aging have tended to disappear."[4] As documented in the preceding chapter and elsewhere, the benefits also extend to the mind and the spirit.

Exercises that best maintain functionality are described as aerobic. For our purposes, aerobic exercises are those that can be continued at a more or less steady pace for a protracted period. The American College of Sports Medicine recommends twenty to sixty minutes of continuous or intermittent activity each day.[5] Aerobic exercise includes such activities as walking, jogging, cross-country skiing, swimming, cycling, dancing, rowing, and rope skipping.

In physiological terms, the energy for these activities is derived from oxidation of glucose and other substances within the muscle fibers themselves. The increased volumes of oxygen are delivered by increased ventilation of the lungs through deeper and more rapid breathing and by increased pumping action of the heart, with a subsequent widening of blood vessels in the active muscles. As fitness improves, the exercise can be speeded up and continued for longer periods. Regular aerobic exercise can be continued into very old age although adjusted in duration and pace as necessary. The American College of Sports Medicine's position on exercise and physical activity for older adults provides a detailed summary of the benefits of exercise for aged individuals and offers guidelines for a comprehensive exercise program.[6]

I would like to point out that aerobic activities are distinguished from those that are intermittent or fluctuating in intensity, such as tennis or basketball. They are also very different from all-out exercises, like the fifty- or hundred-meter dash or even the mile race. In these activities, the muscles contract too quickly to depend on an adequate oxygen supply; therefore, the bulk of the energy requirement is met by nonoxidative chemical reactions in the muscle, such as glycolysis, which is the incomplete breakdown of carbohydrates and the partial release of their available energy. Oxygen debts, which many of us have experienced at various times in our lives, are accumulated during these exercises and are paid off in the recovery period.[7]

Exercises designed to develop muscle strength and muscle mass include weight lifting with free weights, elastic bands, or the resistance of one's own body weight. In addition, one can also work out on weight machines. The benefits of participating in some type of resistance training for aging individuals cannot be emphasized enough. Increases in muscle mass gained through strength training not only enhance the performance of functional tasks and reduce the risk of falls but also improve metabolism, which helps prevent obesity and diabetes. Another benefit of strength training is the prevention of osteoporosis, which is effected through the pull of the muscles on the bone.[8]

Still other kinds of activities, such as golf or bowling, are based more on highly refined skills than on aerobic fitness. My own choices for regular exercise have been, as I have indicated, yoga for flexibility and running, swimming, cross-country skiing, and fast walking for aerobic fitness.

Having discovered cross-country skiing and its indoor version, the NordicTrack, I have discontinued running. Not only is the aerobic demand of cross-country skiing at least equal to that of running, but it has the advantage of exercising the entire body and of being gentler on older joints. I have also found a small hydraulic rowing machine to be effective in maintaining good muscle tone in the entire body. It has become my practice to row briskly for ten minutes before or after skiing (or simulated skiing on the NordicTrack), or after a hike. I swim laps for about thirty minutes at a city recreation center at least once a week in addition to my other regular exercise.

Walking briskly has continued to be my favorite aerobic exercise, and I go for a walk, often in the evening or when I feel myself becoming sleepy over a book, to assimilate what I have just read, to plan a lecture or the next day's work, or to work off an upset. I often walk just to enjoy the scenery, the flowers, or the companionship of my wife.

I would like to offer this caveat: the fitness program I follow is not offered as a model. It's just mine, developed over years and modified from time to time as necessary, desirable, or just for the sake of variety. No doubt, many people in their forties and fifties who are already engaged in an exercise program would find it insufficiently challenging, while many, perhaps most others, in their sixties and older would find it too demanding.

A gentler, general fitness program might include some forms of aerobic exercise that are kinder on the joints than running. The activities I enjoy, such as cross-country skiing, walking, hiking, or swimming, would be good additions for a general program. The advantage of swimming is that it involves virtually every part of the musculoskeletal system while at the same time being easy on old feet, knees, and hip joints. Local YMCA and YWCAs as well as community recreation centers often offer special aquatic exercise programs for older people, the arthritic, and the handicapped. These centers also provide the social support and companionship that often contribute to the enjoyment and success in maintaining an exercise program. However, one should keep in mind that weight-bearing exercises, such as walking, hiking, or cross-country skiing, promote bone strength and, therefore, have a clear advantage over swimming or water aerobics. In addition to aerobic activity, the use of free weights, elastic bands, or a rowing machine to maintain good muscle tone in the entire body would complete a well-rounded fitness regimen of flexibility and aerobic training.

In addition to the physical benefits, regular exercise provides psychological and social benefits. Reported incentives to participate in exercise programs include socialization and pure enjoyment of the activity,[9] as well as the improvement of mood and decreased feelings of depression.[10]

The above examples illustrate various options for comprehensive exercise programs to accommodate a wide range of interests. I encourage those already engaged in regular or even daily exercise programs to continue and even to gradually extend themselves as they find they can. Those who have yet to embark on such a program should begin at a level that is comfortable and pleasant, only gradually increasing the pace and duration of their exertions when they are able. Persons in their later years, especially those who have been sedentary for a long time, should consult with a physical therapist or exercise physiologist after a thorough physical examination by a physician.

In any case, my personal experience, my observation of others, and my studies of the literature strongly suggest that for persons in the middle and later years, walking, which is gradually increased in speed and distance to maintain a challenging level as muscular, respiratory, and circulatory capacities improve, is a highly satisfactory and healthful exercise. An excellent resource, especially for the older person, is *Fitness for Life* by Theodore Berland.[11] This book provides an excellent guide for designing one's own exercise program for flexibility, strength, and endurance. A much briefer guide, *Pep Up Your Life: A Fitness Book for Seniors*, is available through the National Institute on Aging.[12]

BREATHING

Breathing? You may be wondering why I consider a section on breathing to be necessary. "Surely," you might say, "I don't need to be advised to breathe in the same way that I need instruction and encouragement to exercise." You might add, "Surely I don't need instructions on how to breathe any more than I need instructions on how to digest my food; they're both automatic. I leave digestion to my stomach and intestines; they know their business a lot better than I do. Why can't I leave breathing to my lungs?"

The fact is that the lungs do not breathe by themselves; they depend entirely on muscles (there's that musculoskeletal system again!) for their ventilation. The respiratory muscles include the intercostals (between the ribs), the so-called accessory muscles, the diaphragm, and even the abdominal muscles. The attachments of the inspiratory muscles are such that on contraction they raise the ribs, thus expanding the volume of the chest. The expansion of the chest lowers the pressure within, which draws air in through nose or mouth and inflates the lungs. Most inspiratory muscles act by drawing the ribs up and out, much like bucket handles.

The diaphragm acts in quite another way. Between contractions, the relaxed diaphragm is arched upward into the chest, sucked up by the negative pressure (partial vacuum) within the chest. When it contracts, its upward arch is flattened, enlarging the thoracic cavity and drawing air in while compressing the abdominal contents.

The expiratory muscles compress the chest by pulling the ribs down and in, expelling the metabolically altered air that has been heated to body temperature and saturated with water vapor and that contains more carbon dioxide and less oxygen. Under resting conditions, however, most of expiration is accomplished by the elastic recoil of the chest and lungs. The expiratory muscles are called into play when there is need for more rapid and complete expulsion of air in the lungs as in exertion, sneezing, and coughing.

As you can see from the above descriptions, the job of the lungs is largely a passive one. It is a two-way exchange of the metabolic gases (oxygen and carbon dioxide) between air and blood. Contractions and relaxations of the respiratory muscles are ordered and coordinated by nerve centers in the lower parts of the brain. Further, these centers are sensitive to very small changes in the concentration of carbon dioxide in the blood and to impulses from other brain centers and various sensory receptors. Our breathing is automatically adjusted for us according to our changing activities and energy needs; it is even adjusted in anticipation of such changes. Respiration is also automatically involved in and adjusted during such acts as coughing, sneezing, laughing, yawning, swallowing, and the expression of strong emotions (the startled gasp, for example).

The respiratory muscles, like other skeletal muscles, are subject to our conscious and deliberate control. We invoke volitional control when we speak, sing, play wind instruments, swim, blow bubbles, inflate balloons, defecate, or hold our breath for whatever reason. We can also arbitrarily change the rate and depth of respiration at will, up to a point. If we change our blood chemistry too drastically by trying to superimpose our will over automatic control by holding our breath, the body's automatic mechanisms will take over and save us from ourselves.

In addition, any bodily function that is subject to voluntary control is also subject to influence by what we are taught, by our beliefs, and by our assumptions. One unfortunate consequence is that many of us have insidiously and perhaps unconsciously adopted breathing patterns that do not serve us well. The most common of these artifactual patterns suppresses the role of the diaphragm. This, in turn, necessitates compensation by muscles of the rib cage. The adoption of this kind of breathing pattern can, in part, be attributed to the culturally acquired notion that good posture requires that we suck in our guts, stick out our chests, and throw back our shoulders. The result of these incorrect structural adjustments is that the descent of the diaphragm during inhalation, which requires a yielding abdominal wall, is abbreviated. As a result, breathing becomes shallower and, in compensation, more rapid than it need be. Reduced inflation of the lungs renders each breath less effective while at the same time requiring greater expenditures of energy for lifting the chest with each of the more numerous breaths.

Furthermore, we deprive ourselves of the massaging effect that the full rise and fall of the diaphragm has on the abdominal organs. This milking action facilitates venous and lymphatic drainage, which is so necessary for optimal function. Less than desirable patterns of breathing are so deeply embedded in our culture that they are often carried into old age, a time when diaphragmatic breathing is most necessary and long after the abdominal wall has given up the fight and surrendered in permanent protuberance. Observe, if you haven't already, how rapid and shallow the breathing of many old people is, as they move air in and out of only a small portion of the lungs. Every organ, including the brain, suffers from insufficient oxygenation. Also in older people, slouching posture and the stiffening of the chest muscles and rib joints, hastened by inactivity, are also frequent contributors to impaired respiration. Diminished elastic recoil of the lungs, common in older adults, requires increased muscular assistance and is effected at a high energy cost.

At this point, you might ask if old breathing patterns can be unlearned and replaced by new ones. The answer is yes, even in very old persons. It requires only, you guessed it, commitment and disciplined practice. This idea is reminiscent of the anecdote about the mendicant violinist seated on the sidewalk outside Carnegie Hall, his alms cup in front of him. He was approached by a visitor to the city who had difficulty in finding the entrance.

"How do I get into Carnegie Hall, my good man?" the visitor asked.

Stroking the violin strings with emphasis, the musician responded, "Practice, practice, practice!"

I hope you feel ready to start your practice. I think you will find it immensely rewarding if, through the years, you have become a chest-lifting rapid breather. If you have acquired a copy of *Easy Does It Yoga* by Christensen, recommended in chapter 11, you will not need instructions from me. The section of the book that concentrates on breathing is superbly done and includes very helpful illustrations.[13] My own somewhat simpler version of the exercises makes up the sidebar on p. 156.

I want to make it clear that when these breathing exercises are done concurrently with the recommended flexibility exercises, the respiratory muscles become stronger, the lungs more elastic, the rib joints (and the sternum and the spine) more frictionless, and the reserve airspace more capacious. Your happiest surprises, and they are recurrent, will come during your brisker walks or longer runs just as you feel yourself rapidly running out of breath. With a little additional inspiratory effort, you will discover on your very next inhalation that lots of reserve airspace is still available, and you will go sailing over the barrier! Your all-day-long quiet breathing will also benefit from these improvements. Normal breathing will begin to feel almost effortless, and you will find more and more pleasure in the growing abundance of your energy. May you begin to enjoy the same new sense of well-being that began with my first full breath many years ago.

DIET AND WEIGHT CONTROL

I can conceive of no pair of components more fundamental to life, whether the life is that of an amoeba, a whale, or a human being, than those that provide energy: the food we eat, in which energy ultimately derived from the sun is stored, and oxygen, which is essential for the release of that stored (potential) energy. In addition, food is, of course, the source of various materials that, when made available by digestion, are incorporated or converted by cells into their own substances and products. These materials also replenish essential substances that are continually being degraded, used up, or lost to the external environment, such as vitamins, certain amino acids, and minerals.

Having in the previous section dealt with the effective and efficient intake of oxygen, we will now look at diets that best meet the

LEARNING ABDOMINAL DIAPHRAGMATIC BREATHING

First, visualize your chest and abdomen as one large, totally empty sack. The object during each breath is to fill and round out the bottom of the sack first, which automatically draws air into the upper part of the sack. The emptying of the sack is accomplished by its slow collapse during exhalation.

Dress in loose clothing and seat yourself comfortably in a straight chair. Place your hands on your abdomen, fingers widely spread and pointing toward the midline. After an inhalation, exhale slowly through your nose while pressing in firmly on your abdomen with your hands. Next, release the pressure and let your abdomen swell as air is drawn in through the nose. Note the expansion of the chest that automatically and effortlessly follows the bulging of the belly, making room for the full descent of the diaphragm and drawing air into the lungs. The collapse of the belly, with a little assistance from the abdominal muscles, permits the return of the diaphragm to its resting, arched position and is responsible for the expulsion of "stale" air. Repeat this exercise for several minutes, twice each day until the pattern is well established in your mind and in your respiratory muscles. As you practice, think belly out, air in; belly in, air out.

You are now ready to practice abdominal breathing without assistance from your hands. Again, seated in a straight-backed chair or on a stool with your back against a wall, breathe in by letting your abdomen fill. Breathe out by gently and slowly flattening your abdomen. There should be no alternate straightening and rounding of the upper back with each breath. That is, your shoulders should remain in contact with the wall or chair back. Note that your chest seems to go along for the ride, expanding as your lungs fill. Practice this exercise twice daily until it has become automatic and effortless, requiring less and less attention from you.

After mastering these two exercises, you should observe that your breathing has also become slower and slower, a very important sign of improved efficiency. You are now ready for another advance in your breathing exercises. Begin practicing the slow, prolonged expulsion of air until exhalations are at least twice as long as inhalations. This type of breathing allows more efficient transfer of oxygen to the blood and removal of carbon dioxide from the blood, making respiration even more effortless and energy saving.

As your new breathing pattern begins to require less and less attention from you, put it into play not only during your practice periods but in the course of each day while you stand, walk, or engage in other daily activities. Simply tune in to your breathing from time to time and turn on the pattern if it is not yet on automatically.

You may even find this kind of breathing helpful, as I have, in getting to sleep. Lie on your back, bring your knees up, and spread your feet on the bed so that the knees lean on each other. Rest your hands on your abdomen and, focusing on each breath, breathe slowly and deeply. Let a little of your tension evaporate with each exhalation; this produces a letting go that invites sleep.

Congratulate yourself if you have persisted and find yourself breathing diaphragmatically, slowly, and deeply most of the time. You are now ready to call on and enlarge your reserve airspace. Together with your newfound ease of motion, it will make your brisk walks, runs, or other physical activities pure delights. I first want to point out that the quiet breathing described in the preceding paragraphs requires little muscular effort; it is mainly the diaphragm doing all the work. Deep breathing, on the other hand, where the lungs are completely filled with each inhalation and emptied as much as they can be with each exhalation, depends on considerably more muscular effort than quiet breathing. The rib-raising intercostal muscles are very active in deep inhalation as are the so-called accessory respiratory muscles that raise the uppermost ribs. For complete exhalation, the passive recoil of the ribs and diaphragm no longer suffices. Contractions of downward-pulling chest muscles and belly-compressing muscles are required. The compression of the abdomen arches the relaxed diaphragm higher into the chest and causes more effective emptying of the lungs.

To practice what Christensen calls "the complete breath,"* sit up straight, as was previously instructed for the quiet breathing practice. Expel all possible air from the lungs. I say all possible air because negative pressure in the chest prevents the complete collapse of the lungs and total exhalation. Now, relax the abdomen, allowing it to swell as air is drawn into the lungs. When your abdomen is fully expanded, continue to inhale by expanding your chest. You should feel the chest muscles tense. Continue to inhale as the upper chest expands and lifts, filling the lungs to the very top. The abdomen should remain fully expanded and relaxed throughout this process.

Hold the full breath for a moment. Next, let the air out slowly by relaxing and then compressing the rib cage. To complete the expulsion of the stale air, pull in your belly. This will thrust the diaphragm higher in the chest with a piston-like action. Do not lean forward or slouch as you pull the belly in.

Practice this deep breathing exercise for several minutes twice each day. You should progressively increase the volume of air passing in and out of the lungs and gradually prolong the time taken for each breath. Remember that your exhalation time should still be at least twice as long as your inhalation time. Although the full breath requires more muscular effort, the phrase "slow and easy" should reverberate in your head as you do this exercise.

*A. Christensen, *Easy Does It Yoga* (New York: Fireside, 1999).

requirements of the individual healthy life. As with exercise, so much has been published on the subject of nutrition that there is little that I can contribute except to recommend selected sources[14] and to summarize the principles that I think best serve healthful living at all ages. The sources I have suggested show that one need not sacrifice variety or palatability for health.

The energy contained in our food, made available by digestion and released by oxidative and other metabolic processes, is expended in several ways for (1) maintaining the integrity of every cell and the total structure of the organism, in this case the human being; (2) uti-

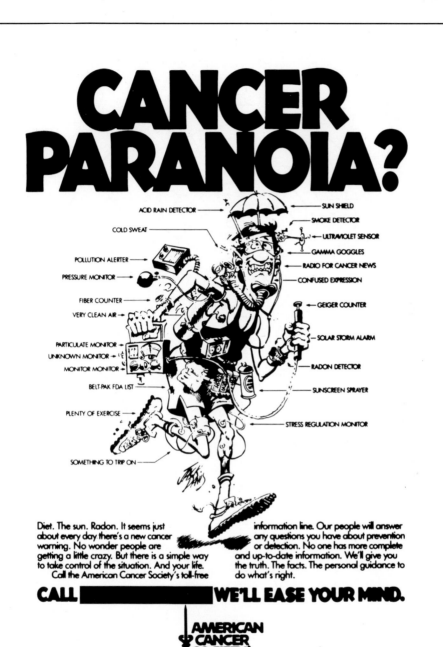

FIGURE 1.

Risk Factor Paranoia

(All images courtesy of the Still National Osteopathic Museum, Kirksville, MO [2004.244.02] and reprinted with permission of the museum.)

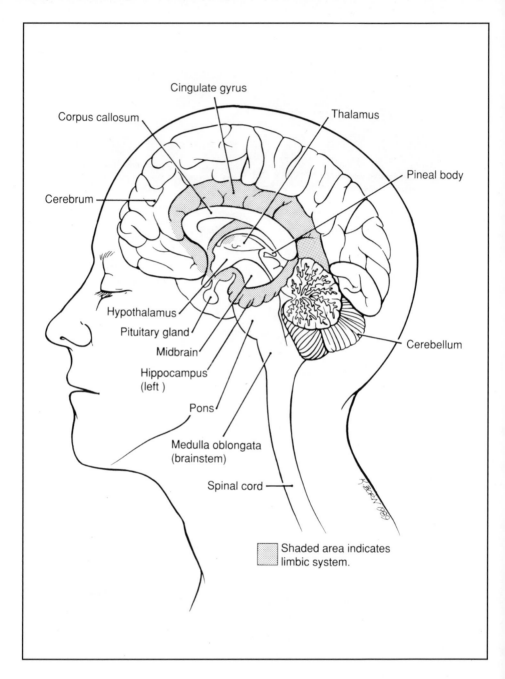

FIGURE 2.
Diagram of the human brain, midline sagittal view.

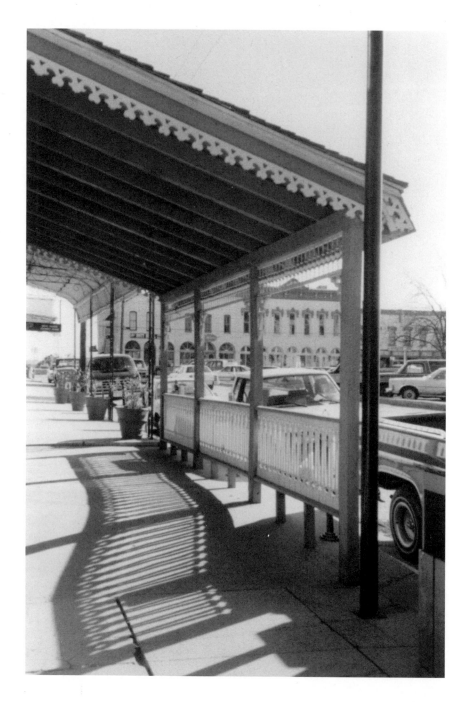

FIGURE 3.
Seemingly straightforward beliefs often cast crooked shadows.

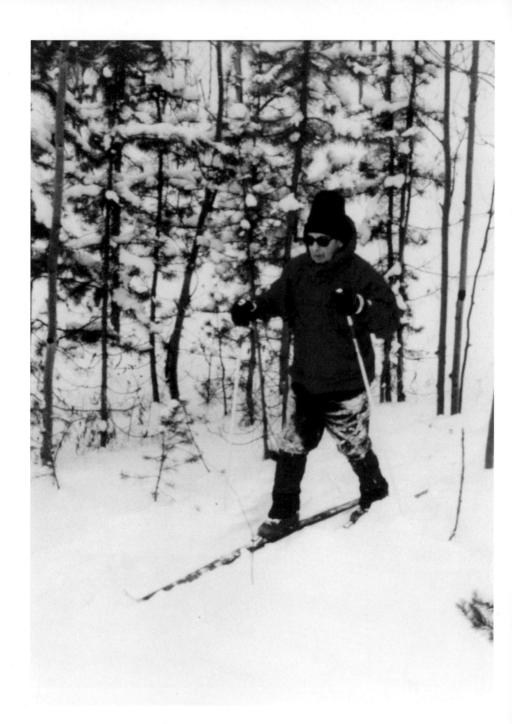

FIGURE 4.
The author on a Colorado ski trail.

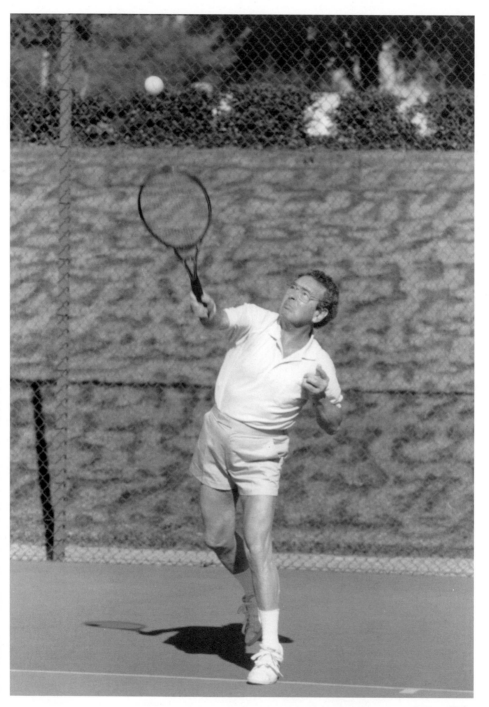

FIGURE 5.
The author, at age 80, on the court.

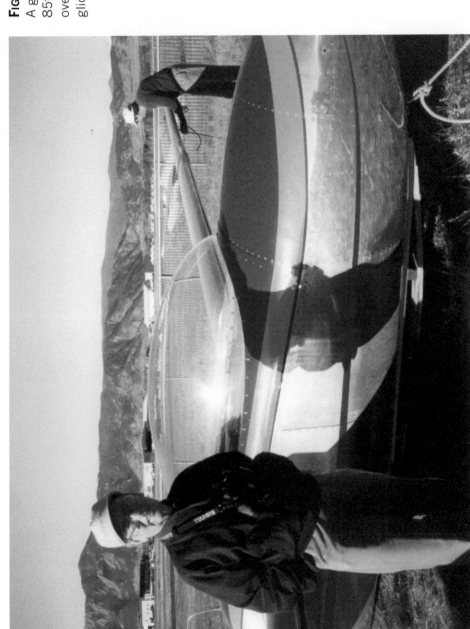

FIGURE 6.
A gift from Jan on my 85th birthday: sailing over the Rockies in a glider.

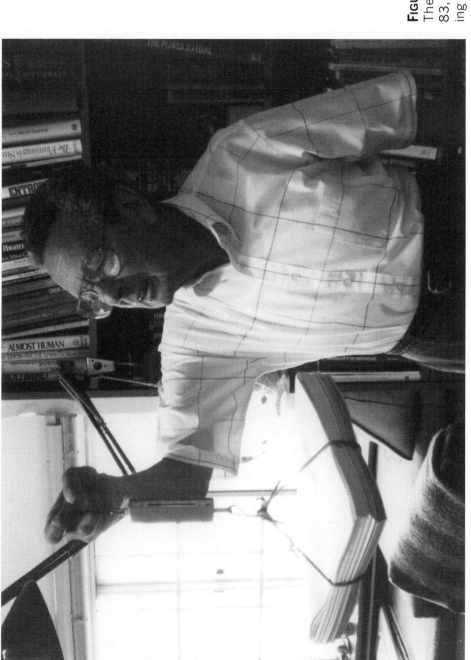

FIGURE 7.
The author, at age 83, carefully weighing his words.

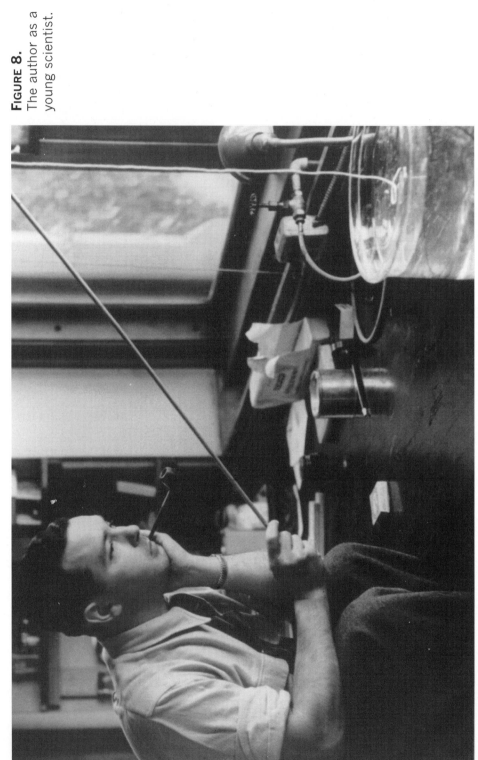

FIGURE 8.
The author as a young scientist.

lizing all the biological mechanisms, such as digestion, circulation, respiration, and brain, nerve, and kidney function; (3) facilitating the activities of the person; and (4) producing heat for maintenance of body temperature.

The first two items add up to the basal metabolic rate, which varies from individual to individual. Energy for exertion and for meeting environmental demand, such as producing more body heat in the cold, is superimposed on basal metabolism. The potential energy contained in our food and expended is measured in the equivalent amount of heat. The measuring unit is the calorie, defined as the amount of heat required to raise the temperature of one milliliter of water by one degree Celsius.

If we take in less food than is required to meet our total energy needs, then the regulatory mechanisms draw on our own tissues to make up the energy deficit. If, on the other hand, we ingest more potential energy than is spent, then the surplus energy is largely converted to more tissue, mainly adipose (fat) tissue.

Thus, we can see that the essence of weight control is the balance between energy spent and energy taken in. Both factors fortunately, or too often unfortunately, are under our personal control—the expenditure of energy over and above basal metabolism through physical exertion and the intake of energy in the form of food consumed. If intake exceeds expenditure, weight increases, mainly by the addition of fat. The reverse is true when the imbalance is in the opposite direction; fat reserves are called on first, thus sparing muscle and other tissues.

Those persons engaged in vigorous athletics or heavy physical labor must have a high caloric intake to balance energy consumption if they are to maintain their weight. Usually, appetites adjust accordingly. Conversely, inactive people must match their caloric intake to their low caloric expenditure. Unfortunately in this instance, their appetites do not always become adjusted automatically and must therefore be controlled voluntarily to avoid a progressive accumulation of fat. Working hard at your desk is not the equivalent of physical labor. Many years ago, a distinguished physiologist measured the difference in energy expenditures between quiet sitting and quiet sitting plus doing difficult mental arithmetic. He concluded that an hour of heavy mental labor could be fueled by half a peanut.

To maintain my weight at a constant level that feels right for me, I long ago adopted the practice of weighing myself almost every morning on the bathroom scale before putting on my clothes. Even a slight increase above my chosen weight (it is almost always an increase!) moves me that very day to adjust either my caloric intake or output, and usually both. However, I have found by experimentation that my weight remains remarkably constant even without monitoring. Thanks to longtime experience, my wife's cooperation, and the automatic regulatory mechanisms in the lower parts of the brain (see chapter 13, "The Body-Minding Brain"), I seem to have struck a reliable balance, and you can, too.

This is not to say that I never stray. I find it especially difficult to control my diet and weight while traveling. I have found that the following equation generally holds true:

$$\text{gracious host} + \text{compliant guest} = \text{fat guest}$$

Just a weekend of indiscretion may require weeks of compensatory discipline on my part.

Readers who have difficulty controlling their weight may wish to consult their physicians, qualified nutritionists, or sources such as those listed at the end of this chapter for guidance in proper diet and exercise. Unfortunately, the curricula of medical schools are notoriously deficient in nutritional instruction, and it may be necessary to seek out certified dietitians or specialists, qualified by virtue of postgraduate training in the field of weight control.

So much for calories and weight control. A detailed review of that subject as well as of nutrition in general is beyond the scope of this book. Again, I will call upon my own experience as a starting point for the reader's own experimentation in this area. My diet is the product of professional study, consultation with nutritionist colleagues, experimentation over many years, and personal taste—my wife's as well as my own.

My diet might be characterized as high in complex carbohydrates and fiber, moderate in protein, and low in fat. (The exaggerated importance attached to high-protein diets in our society is another of our persistent cultural myths.) My carbohydrates and fiber are obtained from vegetables and fruits (both of which, in considerable variety, are a critical component of our daily diet), salads, and whole-grain cereals and breads. Part of the protein component of my diet is derived from moderate portions of poultry, such as chicken and turkey, and fish. I also include nuts and legumes in my diet. As far as possible, my fat intake is limited to polyunsaturated vegetable oils, especially safflower and olive oil. My intake of saturated, high-cholesterol, atherogenic animal fats is reduced to a minimum by severely limiting my consumption of beef and other red meats, butter, whole milk, ice cream, high-fat cheeses, and eggs (no more than two per week). All skin is peeled from chicken and turkey to remove the subcutaneous fat. Fried foods are avoided except occasionally for stir-fried foods done in a thin layer of oil.

My consumption of simple sugars is slight. As one endowed with a very demanding sweet tooth, I have found Rice Dream (made with rice milk), Ice Bean (made with soy beans), sorbet, and low-fat frozen yogurt very satisfying substitutes for ice cream, which is rich in fat and sugar. These and other substitutes for rich sweets, such as carob for chocolate, can be found in most health food stores and, recently, in many supermarkets.

All of my wife's and my home cooking is done without added salt; herbs, spices, or ready-mixed seasonings serve very well in place of salt. Caffeine-containing drinks are also avoided.

As for vitamins, a balanced diet such as mine probably provides all the essential vitamins and minerals I need. However, because my personal consumption of calcium-containing dairy foods is low, I do take a daily mineral supplement and a multivitamin as an extra bit of, probably superfluous, self-assurance. While I would not recommend the practice for those seeking to reduce their weight, my wife and I do occasionally enjoy an alcoholic drink before or with our evening meal.

SUMMARY

Thus, the three other fundamental biological factors that contribute to creating your well-being are exercise, breathing, and nutrition. These, along with freedom of motion, are the fuel that maintains the *vis medicatrix naturae*, or the healer within. Healthful musculoskeletal structure, along with the structure of healthful disciplines, allow for a cascade of benefits to the mind, body, and spirit. That brings me to the topic of our next chapter.

NOTES

1. S. N. Blair et al., "Influences of Cardiorespiratory Fitness and Other Precursors on Cardiovascular Disease and All-Cause Mortality in Men and Women," *Journal of the American Medical Association* 276 (1996): 205–10; M. Gulati et al., "Exercise Capacity and the Risk of Death in Women: The St. James Women Take Heart Project," *Circulation* 108 (2003): 1554–59; L. Myers et al., "Exercise Capacity and Mortality among Men Referred for Exercise Testing," *New England Journal of Medicine* 346 (2002): 793–801.

2. E. Volpi, R. Nazemi, and S. Fujita, "Muscle Tissue Changes with Aging," *Current Opinion in Clinical Nutrition and Metabolic Care* 7 (2004): 405–10.

3. American College of Sports Medicine Position Stand, "Exercise and Physical Activity for Older Adults," *Medicine and Science in Sports and Exercise* 30 (1998): 992–1008.

4. T. F. Williams, "Aging versus Disease," *Generations* (Fall/Winter 1992): 21–25.

5. American College of Sports Medicine and M. H. Whaley, eds., *ACSM's Guidelines for Exercise Testing and Prescription*, 7th ed. (Philadelphia: Lippincott Williams and Wilkins, 2005), pp. 146–47.

6. "Public Resources from ACSM," American College of Sports Medicine, http://www.acsm.org/AM/Template.cfm?Section=General_Public (accessed March 28, 2007).

7. "Exercise: A Guide from the National Institute on Aging," National Institute on Aging, http://www.niapublications.org/exercisebook/exercise book.asp (accessed March 26, 2007).

8. M. E. Nelson, *Strong Women Stay Strong* (New York: Bantam, 1998), p. 41.

9. J. K. Schneider et al., "Exercise Training Program for Older Adults: Incentives and Disincentives for Participation," *Journal of Gerontological Nursing* 29 (2003): 21–31.

10. C. Crowley and H. S. Lodge, *Younger Next Year for Women* (New York: Workman, 2005), pp. 54–56.

11. T. Berland, *Fitness for Life: Exercises for People over 50* (Washington, DC: American Association of Retired Persons, 1986).

12. *Pep Up Your Life: A Fitness Book for Seniors*, AARP in partnership with the President's Council on Physical Fitness and Sports.

13. A. Christensen, *Easy Does It Yoga* (New York: Fireside, 1999).

14. J. Brody, *Jane Brody's Nutrition Book* (New York: Norton, 1981); S. L. Conner and W. E. Conner, *The New American Diet* (New York: Simon and Schuster, 1986); J. D. Goldstritch, *Best Chance Diet* (Atlanta: Humanics, 1982); R. J. Martin, B. D. White, and M. G. Hulsey, "The Regulation of Body Weight," *American Scientist* 79 (1991): 528–41; E. N. Whitney and E. M. N. Hamilton, *Understanding Nutrition*, 2nd ed. (St. Paul, MN: West, 1981); A. Weil and R. Daley, *The Healthy Kitchen* (New York: Knopf, 2002); "American Dietetic Association Home Page," American Dietetic Association, http:// www.eatright.org/cps/rde/xchg/ada/hs.xsl/index.html (accessed March 28, 2007); "Steps to a Healthier You," US Department of Agriculture, http:// www.mypyramid.gov/ (accessed March 28, 2007); "Center for Food Safety & Applied Nutrition," US Food and Drug Administration, http://www .cfsan.fda.gov/ (accessed March 28, 2007); R. L. Duyff and ADA, *American Dietetic Association Complete Food and Nutrition Guide*, 3rd ed. (New York: Wiley, 2006); J. E. Morley, Z. Glick, and L. Z. Rubenstein, *Geriatric Nutrition: A Comprehensive Review*, 2nd ed. (New York: Raven, 1995).

Chapter 13

THE BODY-MINDING BRAIN

"Having accepted and even welcomed my mortality, my quest for completion presents me with new beginnings."

—I. M. Korr

When an organ is mentioned, we almost automatically match it up with a function. For instance, the heart pumps blood, the stomach digests food, the kidney produces urine, and so forth. When we think of the brain, by far the most complex and the second-largest organ in the body, what function usually comes to mind? Precisely that—the mind—and most especially, the human mind and all that *mind* encompasses, such as thought, introspection, reason, language, intellect, imagination, judgment, creativity, empathy, perception, conceptualization, humor, and all our other highly developed mental and emotional capacities. Impalpable though they are, they seem to be viewed as products of the brain very much as insulin is viewed as a product of the pancreas and urine a product of the kidney. Nineteenth-century American writer Ambrose Bierce described mind as "a mysterious form of matter secreted by the brain."[1]

These capacities, most uniquely human, are the business of just a part of the brain and a relatively new part at that. I refer of course to the many-folded, convoluted, lobulated cerebral cortex overlying the rest of the brain, and I especially refer to the most highly evolved part of it, the neocortex. What is more, the rest of the brain, that is, the sub-cortical brain (see figure 2 for its major components), had been in business for hundreds of millions of years before a knowing, thinking, scheming brain began to only recently make its appearance in the course of evolution. What, then, are the functions of the old brain that we have inherited and that have been modified only enough to accom-modate the neocortex and its connections? Collectively, these func-tions can be simply described as "minding the body." I have unashamedly borrowed this phrase from Dr. Joan Borysenko's book *Minding the Body, Mending the Mind*, because it so aptly describes the main, largely unconscious business of the brain.[2]

So, you might ask, what functions am I talking about? First, let me remind you of the homeostatic, protective, regulatory, and recupera-tive processes that form our built-in healthcare system, discussed in chapter 4 as the physician within and the body's own medicines. The brain controls and coordinates all these mechanisms and their utiliza-tion. In presenting the brain's role in the regulation of these mecha-nisms,[3] I shall illustrate with only three—the immune system, tem-perature control, and food intake—and spare you submersion in the ocean of detail in which neurophysiologists delight. However, the principles are very much the same for control of the other functions. My purpose remains to bring what we are reasonably sure of into a coherent health-related perspective.

If you wish to see how these principles operate in other systems, and I hope you do, you will find several more illustrations in appendix 2.

IMMUNE SYSTEM

As is apparently true of all tissues, those that compose the immune system, specifically the bone marrow, thymus, spleen, lymph nodes, and tonsils, are richly supplied with sensory and autonomic nerve fibers. Why sensory nerve fibers, which carry impulses to the central nervous system? Is it not the fibers carrying impulses from the central nervous system that do the regulating? Yes, but in order for the brain centers to control their respective organ functions effectively and precisely, they must have continual feedback from the organs and about the organs. After all, the brain has no way of knowing what is going on in the body or in the external environment except through reports that it receives from out there. These reports come in two forms: (1) as electrical impulses initiated at the sensory endings and receptors and conveyed to the brain centers by chains of neurons (nerve cells) and (2) by chemical or physical changes in the blood. These changes may be in the concentrations of certain substances as simple as carbon dioxide and glucose, or they may be complex substances specific to the organ or tissue. The signal may also be a change in temperature or in osmotic pressure.

The regulatory commands issued by the brain centers to the specific organ or tissue are in the same two forms: impulses and chemical messengers. The impulses originate in the brain centers and are conveyed in descending chains of neurons to the effectors that execute the commands. The final neurons in the chain are either autonomic neurons (innervating glandular, muscular, and vascular components of viscera, endocrine glands, and other organs) or motor neurons controlling contractions and relaxations of skeletal muscles. The chemical messengers include hormones, such as those produced by the pituitary gland (called the master gland because its hormones control secretion by other endocrine glands), and numerous other neurochemicals.

The immune system searches out and destroys or disarms what doesn't belong, what isn't "self." This could be foreign cells, foreign proteins, or even cancer cells. In that function, it has a high degree of autonomy in the quantities and types of defensive cells and immune substances that it produces. Its activities, however, are continually monitored and modulated as necessary by the subcortical, body-minding brain, as it responds in two-way communication to signals and messages from the immune system. Central control becomes especially important during invasion or threat of invasion by foreign organisms or substances.

BODY TEMPERATURE

Variations in body temperature of warm-blooded species (birds and mammals) are ordinarily maintained within narrow limits despite wide fluctuations in environmental temperature and bodily activity. Further, life is certainly impaired, threatened, or terminated by sustained hypo- or hyperthermia.

As was expressed in chapter 4 in the law of fixity—fluxity that operates in homeostasis, temperature is constant or fixed when an influx of heat (heat produced by the body plus any that is absorbed from the environment) is balanced by the outflux (heat lost to the environment). Heat is continually generated by the metabolism and the activities of all the cells. Hence, equal amounts of heat must be continually transferred to the environment if overheating is to be avoided. In this process, heat is lost from the body in the same way that heat is lost from a building by means of infrared radiation to cooler objects, such as walls; convection, which is the warming of moving air; and evaporation from the surface of the body and from the lungs.

Thermoregulatory centers in the hypothalamus (see figure 2) function as the body's thermostats. They are highly sensitive to variations in the temperature of the blood passing through them and to feedback from temperature receptors in the skin and other strategic sources deeper in the body. When an excess of heat production or heat absorption is signaled by a warming of the blood or anticipated by temperature receptors in the skin, the thermoregulatory centers respond by calling for increased heat loss. The two mechanisms are (1) the shunting of blood from inside the body to the surface to accelerate radiation and convection and (2) the production of adequate quantities of water that then become available for evaporation from the surface.

The first method is achieved by dilating blood vessels in the skin (through sympathetic nerve fibers) and the second by stimulating sweat gland secretion (also through their sympathetic innervation).

Conversely, when blood temperature drops, reflecting an excess of heat loss, the brain centers call for constriction of blood vessels in the skin and dilatation elsewhere, which shifts blood from the surface to deeper tissues, and for cessation of sweating. When these efforts at conservation of heat do not suffice and blood temperature continues to drop, then heat production is turned up. In this instance, the brain centers via motor pathways call for increased muscular tension and active shivering, which rapidly generates large amounts of heat that warms the blood.

As when fever occurs, the hypothalamic thermostats can be, and often are, reset. With fever, the brain's thermostats have been reset to a higher temperature. I would like to point out that fever is one of the body's adaptive defense mechanisms against infection and should not be interfered with unless the temperature rises to dangerous levels. Further, there is reason for concern about the defensive and recuperative resources of a patient whose temperature remains unelevated during a serious infection.

FOOD INTAKE

Food intake is controlled by two hypothalamic centers—an appetite center, which directs the animal to eat, and a satiety center, which signals "enough." One signal to seek food (what we experience as hunger) is apparently initiated by a drop in blood sugar and may subsequently be reinforced by contractions of the stomach (hunger pangs), among other signals. Since satiety occurs long before the food has been digested, absorbed, and assimilated, some other signal seems to be involved in this process, perhaps distention of the stomach.

It is also important to remember that eating includes the complex processes of chewing and swallowing; both of which are organized and coordinated by subcortical parts of the brain. Still, other brain centers are involved in such corrective, defensive, and highly coordinated processes as vomiting, coughing, and sneezing.

CONTROL OF POSTURE, EQUILIBRIUM, AND MOTOR AND BEHAVIORAL PATTERNS

Having completed my discussion of the three mechanisms—the immune system, body temperature, and food intake, which the brain regulates in its function as the physician within—I would like to turn to another function. As we sit, stand, walk, or run, our body weight is supported by precisely adjusted tensions of muscles (the extensors) that keep the knees, hips, and spine from collapsing under the force of gravity. Continual adjustments of contractions of these postural, weight-supporting muscles is done without thought for us by various reflex mechanisms in the spinal cord, brain stem, cerebellum, and other subcortical brain centers (see figure 2). These adjustments are in response to continual streams of impulses from receptors in the muscles, tendons, ligaments, and joints and even pressure receptors in the feet. Similar principles and mechanisms operate in maintaining and restoring our balance or equilibrium. They permit us to move and change the configuration of our bodies without falling over as we bend forward, extend our arms, or move our heads in one way or another; walk or run; abruptly change directions; and so forth. As the distinguished orthopedist Dr. Arthur Steindler wrote many years ago, "Walking, for man, is a series of catastrophes, narrowly averted."[4]

Thus, every step incurs momentary imbalance as one foot is raised for the next forward step and as the center of gravity, approximately at the level of the navel, moves precariously forward of the supporting foot. Ordinarily, the maintenance and restoration of balance as we stand or move requires no thought or conscious attention. We take them for granted, thanks to the cerebellum and other centers in the hindbrain and midbrain. However, for the maintenance of our equilibrium, these centers require more than continual reporting from muscles, tendons, ligaments, and joints. Of special importance in maintaining and recovering our balance are the labyrinths in the inner ears, receptors in ligaments of the upper neck that report the orientation of the head with respect to the body, and of course the eyes. Together, these three things keep the brain centers, and us, apprised of our moment-to-moment orientation in space and of the direction of our movement. When the various receptors and sensory organs send in conflicting reports about our orientation in space, as often happens on the high seas, the body-minding brain sort of throws up its hands—and then we throw up!

Again, the same principles of control by the body-minding brain apply as we look into even more complex motor patterns. Whatever the motion we choose to carry out from moment to moment, the cortex delegates responsibility for organizing countless component mechanisms to lower centers in the brain and spinal cord. This is true whether the motion is the simple act of extending an arm, turning the head, or walking; this even includes the painfully learned, long-practiced, and highly refined skills that are involved, for example, in playing a musical instrument.

When the cortex calls for a particular motion, it does not call on individual muscles (it doesn't even know their names!) to instruct each one from millisecond to millisecond about the force, extent, or speed of contraction and the timing, rate, and degree of relaxation. The cortex merely decides each moment what movement it wants (actually, the person decides) and relies on the subordinate centers to organize and orchestrate it.

What, then, is the purpose of practice? Why the long hours to develop and train our bodies to perform specific skills and tasks? Through practice, the cortex learns and remembers how to communicate the requests to the lower centers that will produce the desired result. At the same time that the cortex concentrates on what, for example, it wants the little finger of the left hand to do on the keyboard, it also relies on the lower centers, as we have seen, to maintain flexible, compliant body support and to keep the body from falling over as its weight shifts on the piano bench from one buttock to the other.

We turn now to a still-higher order of complexity, that of survival-related, emotion-based behavior patterns that are also largely organized in the ancient body-minding brain. Imagine a hungry, male, carnivorous animal resting on a rock or a fallen tree trunk in the forest. He suddenly catches scent or sight of another animal in the vicinity. Arousal centers in the brain alert the animal for possible action. But what kind of action? Wordless questions might arise in the animal's mind: Is it a receptive female of my species? Is it my next meal, on foot? Does it have designs on me as its next meal? Is it an adversary seeking to challenge me to a duel for food or a mate? Is it nothing that concerns me? Of course, there really isn't time to ask all these questions if the animal is to survive and have its way. They seem to be instantaneously asked and answered, yes or no. Nevertheless, the questions represent most of the possibilities.

The answers to the above questions elicit from the limbic system (see figure 2), in the most modern part of the body-minding brain, the appropriate emotion, whether it be sexual arousal, fear, rage, and so on. (By appropriate emotion, I mean that which prompts the bodily response most adaptive to the objective situation and that favors survival of the individual and of the species.) It then elicits the appropriate motor patterns in all their enormous complexity, such as courting and copulation, fight, flight, or pursuit. Finally, it prompts the appropriate changes in circulation, respiration, and metabolism.

These primitive, life-preserving emotions and behavioral and autonomic patterns are part of our evolutionary legacy. They and the other body-minding functions of the brain have served humans for tens of millions of years and have made possible the emergence and survival of the species. As discussed in chapter 8, we humans use them, however, in ways and in circumstances that are vastly different from those in which they evolved and from those in which they continue to be used in the wild.

Our individual levels of health depend crucially on how we use and abuse the body-minding brain in our daily lives. I very sincerely hope it has become clear from this chapter that this part of the brain is the most dominant, pervasive, and reliable coronet of our personal healthcare systems. Many years ago, the famous Harvard physiologist Walter B. Cannon wrote a provocative little book on the subject of homeostasis (the word he coined), which he titled *Wisdom of the Body*.[5] Much of that wisdom resides in the body-minding brain. How well it serves each of us depends, as it does with respect to all other organs, on what I have called the context that each of us provides for its functioning. In short, it depends on what the cerebral cortex hath wrought. This will be the subject of my next chapter.

NOTES

1. A. Bierce, *The Devil's Dictionary* (Mount Vernon, NY: Peter Pauper, 1958).

2. J. Borysenko, *Minding the Body, Mending the Mind* (Reading, MA: Addison-Wesley, 1987).

3. R. E. Ornstein and D. Sobel, *The Healing Brain* (New York: Simon and Schuster, 1987).

4. A. Steindler, "The Classic: Osteoporosis 1956," *Clinical Orthopaedics and Related Research* 443 (2006): 3–9, discussion 2.

5. W. B. Cannon, *Wisdom of the Body* (Gloucester, MA: Peter Smith, 1963).

Chapter 14

THE MIND-MINDING PERSON

"The more I learn, the less I have to remember. The less the need to remember, the larger the space for learning."

—I. M. Korr

THE MEETING OF THE OLD AND THE NEW

How is the body-minding brain affected by the superimposition of the human neocortex? Are the functions of the body-minding brain significantly altered by the impulses and neurochemicals showered upon it by the neocortex? As we have seen, the neocortex calls on and relies on these "lower" centers to mobilize the body mechanisms that will execute its commands.

Having, in effect, been placed in command of the wonderfully reliable old mechanisms that were the subject of the preceding chapter, the human neocortex, a relative newcomer, is presented with the enormous challenge of learning to use these mechanisms in ways that best serve human lives and human goals. Further, it must do so within the unavoidable limits set by the primeval origins of these mechanisms that evolved in animals that lived incomparably simpler lives in environments not subject, as they are today, to change by human intervention. Therefore, the neocortex must not ask them to do what they cannot do or to do what they can do for too long in the wrong way. Such conflicting messages would impair the body-minding ability of the older mechanisms, with consequences extending to the brain itself.

In describing the impact of evolution on human development in chapters 8 and 9, I illustrated the harmful demands that we humans often place on these mechanisms. Biomedical literature is replete with reports on psychogenic factors in heart disease, cancer, stroke, hypertension, peptic ulcers, arthritis, obesity, and impaired immunity, to name just a few examples. Psychoneuroimmunology is but one of the more recent research areas to appear on the psychosomatic scene, and the pathogenic impact of unphysiologic, antihomeostatic demands made by the neocortex has been reported in thousands of scientific and clinical publications in many languages. However, I will not dwell on these research areas since the focus of this book remains less on diseases and their causes than on the avoidance of disease. Once again, I am specifically focusing on high-level health and *its* causes.

When I think of the "old" and the "new" parts of the brain, I imagine a sophisticated neocortex that feels hampered and frustrated by the limitations of the old-fashioned machinery as it impatiently seeks to drive that "clunker" beyond its limits. Is this a characteristic of the generic human neocortex? Must we wait for the evolutionary process either to modernize the body-minding brain to meet cortical demands or to create a neocortex more moderate in its demands? No, this does not characterize the human neocortex. Millions of men and women achieve their goals, often lofty, exacting goals, for which they are honored and thanked by their contemporaries and by posterity. In addition, these individuals continue to strive into their seventies, eighties, and beyond in good and even excellent health. We have much to learn from them.

MAKING PEACE BETWEEN THE OLD AND THE NEW

If we are to improve personal, national, and even world health and thereby reduce the burden of disease, we must learn what we can from those who are, or have been, enduringly healthy though severely challenged. We must also consider how the cerebral hemispheres of the remaining tens and hundreds of millions are to be coached in the more successful utilization of their subjacent body-minding brains. Is there anything that each of us can call on to do that job? Yes, there is. And in this we are confronted by one of the most profound, perplexing, enduring, and possibly unsolvable mysteries of life. This mystery has engaged philosophers and poets for thousands of years and, more recently, such distinguished Nobel laureate neuroscientists as John C. Eccles and Roger W. Sperry. The mystery I speak of is the mind and its relation to the brain.

THE BRAIN-MIND QUESTION

I do not pretend that what I have to offer at last solves the mystery or even that it is very original, but only that it has a rational basis (for which the human mind hungers) and that it is consistent with, though more intricate than, other natural phenomena.

You may recall the principle of interactive unity, or the oneness of the person, discussed in chapter 2. To review, I explained how organized totalities are different from and more than the sum of their parts; new qualities emerge at each higher level of organization that cannot be accounted for by the properties of the components. These properties are not necessarily reflected in the emergent qualities or phenomena. I offered three examples: (1) Although water molecules consist of two hydrogen atoms and one oxygen atom, their properties are not evident in the properties of any of the three states of water (solid, liquid, and gas). (2) Similarly, the nature of a bee colony cannot be disclosed by studying individual bees. (3) Finally, traffic patterns cannot be predicted from observations of individual cars and drivers. Yet there is no denying that the emergent phenomenon or quality in each example is a product of components assembled in certain interrelational configurations.

The principle summarized and illustrated in the foregoing paragraph is the kind of unprovable generalization that often illuminates the scientist's life. After all, the scientist's lifelong quest is for order, parsimony, and unity and to discover connections among apparently disparate, unordered, scattered, unconnected things and events. The value of such generalizations to the scientist is not only in the satisfaction and joy that they bring, but in the fact that they open up new questions for investigation. I have found great excitement in the awareness that the principle that explains the emergence of water, bee colonies, traffic jams, human society, and much else from their respective components also applies to the mind, for mind, too, is an emergent phenomenon.

When approximately one hundred billion neurons of many types, their countless and changing synaptic interconnections, the chemicals they secrete, and various non-neuronal cells are organized into a human cortex-rich brain, a new phenomenon emerges—the mind. Just as we cannot discuss the viscosity, surface tension, freezing and boiling points, and other properties of water in terms that also describe the physicochemical properties of hydrogen and oxygen, so we cannot describe thought, feelings, imagination, or consciousness in bioelectric and neurochemical terms. This is true even though mental events may be correlated in various ways with bioelectric and neurochemical phenomena as revealed by such technologies as magnetic resonance imaging, just as water is correlated with two-to-one bonding of hydrogen and oxygen. It is nice to know that water is composed of hydrogen and oxygen in certain interrelational configurations, but that knowledge does not *explain* water. In the same way, it is good to know that the appetite center, for example, in response to certain incoming impulses fires impulses that you, in turn, experience as hunger. However, the translation of objective bioelectric impulses into the subjective sensation of hunger remains beyond our comprehension. As another example, we cannot explain how impulses that originate in your retina and evoke bioelectric responses in the visual cortex are translated into what you see (the image of a mountain, a flower, or another person), nor do we understand how the perception of beauty, the recognition of the person, or the feeling of pleasure that you may experience is created.

As a matter of fact, neuroscience has not been able to explain the comparatively simple visual component that preceded and elicited the perceptions, thoughts, and feelings described above. For example, one unanswered and perhaps unanswerable question is how does the brain, given the two-dimensional impulse patterns presented to it by the retina(s), convert them to the three-dimensional vision that we take for granted?

Perhaps more difficult is the question of how the brain summons to the mind's eye scenes, objects, and faces seen a day, a month, or many years ago. Even more mysterious, how does it form and project previously unseen images as in fantasy and dreams and in artistic creation? Where is the film stored? Where is the projector, and where is the screen?

THE LEAP FROM BRAIN TO MIND

The leap from the objective neurobiologic to the subjective mental and emotional survey crosses a wide chasm between two very different terrains. The chasm is in our understanding and not in nature. The questions of whether, when, and how the chasm is to be traversed and intelligible communication begun between the two territories will continue to engage scientists and practitioners, as well as philosophers and poets, for decades to come. It occurs to me to suggest that "spirit" is often invoked to bridge the gap in our understanding between the objective biophysical phenomena that are demonstrable to others and the private, subjective experience.

WHAT OR WHO IS IN CHARGE?

There is another parallel between mind and other emergent phenomena, one with enormously exciting implications. I refer to the dominating influence of the emergent entity on its own components. Hydrogen and oxygen, having joined to form water, are then constrained in their behavior by the properties of water in each of its three states. Individual bees, while continuing to behave like bees, are nevertheless governed by the laws of the society they form. So, too, the movement of individual cars is in accordance with the traffic patterns that they collectively form. Similarly, the mind emerges from the activities of neuronal networks, while from moment to moment assigning those networks and their neuronal components their tasks. In doing so, the mind governs the brain and its billions of neurons, of which, at the same time, it is evidently the product.

How are tasks chosen? According to what criteria are goals and objectives chosen? Before responding to these questions, let us recall another leap already taken and the chasm that we crossed in that leap. In chapter 2 on interactive unity, I tried to show the functional inseparability and the unity of body and mind, which I symbolized as bodymind. Clearly, the unifying link is the brain, which is both a part of the body in two-way communication with every part of it and, apparently, the physical source of each mind.

What was the chasm over which we leaped? In the discussion of interactive unity, I stated that, while body and mind in their interrelational configuration appear to compose the person, the person (or if you prefer, the self) is far more than their sum (another emergent phenomenon). The person, initially the genetic product of prior generations and of intrauterine development, is also the product of his or her entire history, recorded and reflected in the bodymind. Guided by criteria, goals, and objectives accumulated, modified, and sifted during his or her history, the person is, whether willing or competent, in charge of his or her mind and, hence, of bodymind.

Nowhere is awareness of this power more eloquently expressed than in the familiar assertions, "I made up my mind," "I changed my mind," and "I put my mind to work." That power is perhaps more elegantly expressed, as the uniquely human one that it is, in a statement given by behavioral scientist Sarah B. Hrdy in 1983: "The behavior of animals is determined mostly by evolution, while humans have options for self-improvement in line with their civilized ideals."

The challenge to each of us, then, is to rearrange, change, or make up our minds in such ways that we can better serve our civilized ideals. Further, this must be accomplished at no cost to health and well-being.

PSYCHOLOGICAL CAUSES OF DISEASE

As is true in other aspects of medical thought and practice, the usual emphasis in this area is also on risk factors contributing to various specific diseases and organ failures. However, these risk factors are in the psychological domain and are dubbed psychosocial, psychoemotional, psychogenic, psychosomatic, or some other term according to one's preference. Thus anger and hostility are seen as contributing to heart disease, feelings of helplessness to cancer, stress to ulcers or arthritis, anxiety to hypertension, and so forth. There can be no doubt, of course, that avoidance or moderation of risk factors is desirable, whether they be physical, such as smoking, or whether they be psychological.

I emphasize again that there are no single causes, that there are multiple factors implicated in the etiology or causation of each illness, and that we still do not know why some or even most of those who indulge in or are exposed to known risk factors do not succumb to the predicted diseases. As with the majority of students in my freshman classes and with HIV survivors, it would be nice to know their secret advantages. What is it that defends us so successfully against potent risk factors, whether they are physical (somatic) or psychological?

The strategy of risk factor appraisal and avoidance unquestionably has had preventive value, reflected most notably in the reduced incidence of heart disease. Nevertheless, I have long felt that the focus on individual risk factors and their statistically significant effects, with the accompanying lists of injunctions and prohibitions, is essentially a negative and forbidding approach. It is reminiscent of the wise advice offered by the great and long-playing baseball pitcher Satchel Paige: "Don't look back. Something might be gaining on you."[1] The risk-factor approach is one of continual, often fearful, vigilance, looking back for something that might be gaining on us.

PSYCHOLOGICAL CAUSES OF HEALTH

If some kinds of thoughts, feelings, attitudes, perceptions, and responses can contribute to illness, then certainly there must be other kinds that favor recovery from illnesses and that even prevent illness by contributing to higher levels of health.

What is needed is a much more positive strategy, the focus of which is on the factors that move us to higher levels on the health continuum. After all, the higher the level of health, the less the potency of risk factors and the less our vulnerability to disease in general.

In the next chapter, on changing the mind, we need to identify the attitudes, behaviors, feelings, perceptions, beliefs, responses, and interpersonal relationships that move us to the brighter hues on the health spectrum, whatever our age, rather than focusing on the sins of self-abuse and their penalties. Let us focus more on the positive rewards rather than on the negative consequences.

A cogent demonstration of the empowering influence of the mind on the body's healthcare system is the so-called placebo effect, which for reasons that will become obvious should more correctly be designated as the placebo response.[2] *Placebo* is a Latin word meaning "I will please." In clinical trials designed, for example, to test the efficacy of a medication, a placebo is given to patients in the nontreatment or control group. It is similar in appearance and taste to the medication being tested. Double-blinded studies minimize statistical errors due to spontaneous recovery and to investigator bias by administering the real treatment to one group of patients (the experimental group) and the placebo to a comparable and similarly afflicted control group, without the investigator or the patient knowing which has been administered.

Assessment of the placebo effect is necessitated by the consistent observation in thousands of clinical trials that a sizable portion, often as large as one-third and even one-half, of the control group who have not received the medication or treatment have nevertheless recovered or improved. The placebo effect, therefore, is regarded as a nuisance and a source of error for which statistical correction must be made if the efficacy of the real treatment is to be accurately assessed.

Overlooked from this viewpoint is the vital fact that these spontaneous recoveries and improvements are manifestations of the potency of the patient's own healthcare system and its internal medicines. In addition, one must consider that these may have been potentiated and triggered into action by the patient's thoughts, perceptions, and feelings, whether hope, expectations, optimism, desire to please the doctor, confidence in self or doctor, beliefs about the illness or the treatment, determination, or even desperation after having tried everything else (that is, the patient thinks, "This has got to work!").

This is the essential message cited in books such as those of Norman Cousins, in which he describes his own remarkable recoveries from incurable and life-threatening diseases.[3] It is also the basis for Cousins's remark that "The two most neglected systems in the practice of medicine are the closely connected belief system and healing system," and for his advice that "While you may have to accept the diagnosis, you don't have to accept the prognosis; you have more control over that than you've been taught to believe." In *Love, Medicine and Miracles*, surgeon Bernie Siegel describes how, by his own behavior with his cancer patients, he deliberately attempts to activate their powers of healing and guides them to do the same for themselves.[4] Other books, such as those by Blair Justice, Joan Borysenko, Deepak Chopra, Kenneth Pelletier, Jeanne Achterberg, and Martin L. Rossman, collectively present overwhelming evidence for healing, recuperation, restoration of health, and prolongation of life through appropriate changes in patient beliefs, attitudes, expectations, and subsequent behaviors and feelings.[5]

Many studies, both prospective and retrospective, on large numbers of seriously or terminally ill patients have validated the advice given by the authors in the previous paragraph and have demonstrated the crucial importance of the patient's attitudes and perceptions to clinical outcome and survival, often to the bafflement of the specialists and statisticians.[6]

Hence, what is a nuisance and a source of error from one viewpoint is an essence and a source of welcome outcomes from another. The latter viewpoint must guide more and more the teaching and the practice of medicine, and the physician's aim must more and more become that of evoking and empowering the patient's own recuperative powers.[7]

The object, in short, is to learn how and to teach others how to consciously turn on and keep turned on the placebo response, or the bodymind's health-maintaining and health-restoring powers. These powers are indeed the essence and the source of healing. Until the healing professions and their educational systems assume their share of the responsibility, turning on will remain your responsibility and mine.

In summary, I would like to say that it is most encouraging to witness the flourishing of organizations, journals, books, and television programs on the healing and health-enhancing powers of the mind.[8] For the most part, these have been relegated to the realm of alternative medicine. It is to the enormous credit of the National Institutes of Health that the National Center for Complementary and Alternative Medicine was established to promote and support research in these unorthodox practices. It is also noteworthy that these unconventional therapies are in widespread and increasing use as has been documented in several studies and consumer reports. See, for example, a report in the *New England Journal of Medicine*.[9] The many references cited at the end of this chapter can be used as resources and applied to the *changing of the mind*, the subject of our next chapter.

NOTES

1. L. "Satchel" Paige, *Maybe I'll Pitch Forever* (New York: Doubleday, 2000).

2. H. A. Guess et al., eds., *The Science of the Placebo: Toward an Interdisciplinary Research Agenda* (London: BMJ Books, 2002); A. Hrøbjartssøn and P. C. Gøtzsche, "Is the Placebo Powerless? An Analysis of Clinical Trials Comparing Placebo with No Treatment," *New England Journal of Medicine* 344 (2001): 1594–1602; T. Kaptchuk and M. Croucher, *The Healing Arts: Exploring the Medical Ways of the World* (New York: Summit, 1987); A. F. Leuchter et al., "Changes in Brain Function of Depressed Subjects during Treatment with Placebo," *American Journal of Psychiatry* 159 (2002): 122–29; G. Montgomery and I. Kirsch, "Classical Conditioning and the Placebo Effect," *Pain* 72 (1997): 107–13; H. Brody and D. Brody, *The Placebo Response* (New York: HarperCollins, 1997).

3. N. Cousins, *Anatomy of an Illness as Perceived by the Patient* (New York: Norton, 1979); N. Cousins, *The Healing Heart* (New York: Norton, 1983).

4. B. S. Siegel, *Love, Medicine and Miracles* (New York: Harper and Row, 1986).

5. J. Achterberg, *Imagery in Healing: Shamanism and Modern Medicine* (Boston: New Science Library, 1985); J. Borysenko, *Minding the Body, Mending the Mind* (Reading, MA: Addison-Wesley, 1987); D. Chopra, *Quantum Healing: Exploring the Frontiers of Mind/Body Medicine* (New York: Bantam, 1989); D. Chopra, *Perfect Health* (New York: Three Rivers Press, 2000); B. Justice, *Who Gets Sick: Thinking and Health* (Houston: Peak Press, 1987); K. R. Pelletier, *Mind as Healer, Mind as Slayer: A Holistic Approach to Preventing Stress Disorders* (New York: Delta, 1977); M. L. Rossman, *Healing Yourself* (New York: Walker, 1987).

6. C. Hirshberg and M. I. Barasch, *Remarkable Recovery: What Extraordinary Healings Tell Us about Getting Well and Staying Well* (New York: Riverhead, 1995).

7. H. Brody and D. Brody, *The Placebo Response* (New York: Cliff Street, 2000).

8. G. Harris, *Body and Soul* (New York: Kensington, 1999).

9. D. M. Eisenberg et al., "Unconventional Medicine in the United States: Prevalence, Costs, and Patterns of Use," *New England Journal of Medicine* 328 (1993): 246–52.

Chapter 15

CHANGING THE MIND

"The less certain I become about what is right or wrong, virtuous or evil, good or bad for others, the more certain I become about what is right for me."

—I. M. Korr

THE MIND-SET OF MY FIRST FORTY-PLUS YEARS

In keeping with the central theme of this book, I would like now to impress on my readers that the very principles that operate in *cures*, *spontaneous remissions*, and *miraculous recoveries* also operate in spontaneous prevention of disease through the enhancement of health. These health-enhancing, preventive attitudes, behaviors, perceptions, and responses can be learned, as I can attest from my own experiences in the second half of my life. I hope that I may again be forgiven for drawing on my own experiences. Largely anecdotal, they are offered, not as proof of the principles that I embrace, by which I live, and that I recommend, but as an illustration of these principles. Further, they are principles that are being more and more firmly established by the researchers and clinicians cited later in this chapter. In describing what I learned from my experiences, it is my hope that these lessons will help my readers, their children, and their children's children to get off to a much earlier start in healthful living.

My first forty-plus years produced a man who at this point seems so remote and different from me now that I often find myself thinking of him in the third person. I nevertheless feel a deep sympathy for him because there was so much of the joy of living that he—that is, I—had missed and, what is even sadder, without knowing what I was missing. I seem to have been driven by a need for approval and acknowledgment. The underlying need, I am convinced, was for self-approval. Pressed on by my expectation of an early demise, I lived in a relentless hurry, seeking to build a creditable record of accomplishment before my time ran out.

Depending as I did not only on my own work but also on the contributions of those who served as teachers and researchers in the department I chaired, I made sure that they felt my impatience. Knowing a little about dose-related effects, I have often wondered whether it was more than coincidence that the seven persons who died during and after my administration did so in the order in which they were appointed.

Impatient, hypercritical, and demanding, I often dashed off critical memos to administrators. I habitually chided other department heads, whom I viewed as my competitors for recognition and the budget dollar, for placing departmental turf interests above those of the medical college. Having developed what was, in my judgment, a clear and absolutely perfect vision of the needed changes in curriculum, research, and college policies, I lived in resentment of and anger at those whom I perceived to be standing in the way. I often found myself wishing they would, in one way or another, get out of the way so that we could make some progress toward the goals I proposed—goals that they, of course, were too benighted to appreciate! While the quality of my work and that of the division received its due recognition, so did my abrasiveness: I came to be known at the medical college as

Carborundum Korr. Given my competitiveness, hostility, irascibility, and pressing sense of urgency, I certainly would have qualified for what is today known as the type A personality, with all of its known hazards to health.

My anger extended to inanimate objects as well. I often found myself flying into a rage at some recalcitrant, uncooperative piece of laboratory equipment; an instrument; or a home appliance. Sometimes these instances resulted in destruction to myself, to the object, or both. I remember one incident that amused my dining companions but that only caused me embarrassment and smarting thighs. As I raised a full coffee cup to my lips, I carelessly spilled some on my light-gray trousers. In quick anger, I set the cup down with a bang, causing more spillage, painful burns to myself, and further damage to my clothing, as I exclaimed, "Damn splashy coffee!"

During the preceding years, I had consciously or unconsciously adopted certain rigid, binding rules of behavior and expected others under my influence to rigorously avoid overstepping the lines that separated my conceptions of right and wrong. My principles of behavior included a sharp distinction, of which I of course was the sole arbiter, between proper, uplifting, and educational recreation on the one hand and between frivolous wastes of time and money on the other. As a result, I deprived my son and myself of many pleasures we might have shared as he was growing up, such as those of fishing, camping, boating, attending sporting events, or just loafing. I also deprived my collaborators and myself of the comradeship that would have made a joy of our work rather than a compulsion.

Under that bristling armor lived a timorous, diffident, uncertain man who, by his acts of aggressiveness, sought desperately to find a reason to approve of himself and whose greatest pleasure was in proving himself right and, failing that, proving others wrong.

THE BEGINNING OF MIND-CHANGE

In chapter 1, I described my personal saga and the profound changes in feelings, behaviors, interests, personal relationships, responses, and activities that overall composed changes in my personality that I (and those around me) began to enjoy in my second forty-year period and that I still enjoy. A rereading of that part of the chapter did, however, remind me of the remarkable and very welcome degree to which mindset and ways of being and becoming can be changed. Perhaps the most palpable change in my later years is that the more my time runs out, the less hurried I am.

My hardiness, which I will explain later, was manifested in the fact that I remained in excellent health during and following what was the most tragic period of my life, a time in which bereavements and life changes said to be the most stressful and health-damaging dominated my life.[1] Between sixty-six and sixty-eight, I suffered the death of my wife of thirty-six years and of three longtime colleagues who had become very dear to me. In that same period, I retired from the Kirksville College of Osteopathic Medicine in rural Missouri and moved to Michigan State University, located in a vastly different physical and cultural environment. In Michigan, I undertook very different responsibilities with a new team of colleagues while adjusting to single life.

In the remainder of this chapter, I intend to identify some factors that contributed to the dramatic change in how I experienced and dealt with the world. I have no doubt that the most crucial factor, which was initiated and facilitated by increased bodily flexibility, was the reflected increase in behavioral flexibility. My armor of tight muscles and muscle-compressed stiff joints gradually melted away, and with this came the relinquishing of old, rigid patterns of behavior and their replacement by freer, more adaptive ones. As the bombardment of my brain by repetitive streams of uninterpretable impulses from my tense body gradually subsided, my ever-present feelings of tension began to yield to longer and longer periods of quietude and relaxation.

With the gradual dropping away of my armor, more and more of *me* came into view for scrutiny. And scrutinize I did, seeking with growing avidity self-knowledge and understanding. An aversive response to some disturbing circumstance or to the word or deed of another person began, with increasing promptness, to raise questions in my mind about the appropriateness of my response. I discovered that in the very process of questioning the validity and the justification for my ire and acrimony, for example, they evaporated without residue.

LEARNING FROM OTHERS

I began to listen with new interest even to casual remarks about me by others for whatever helpful hints I might find in them. Several of these have remained firmly recorded in my memory. At first painful, each little insight produced a flash of self-knowledge. As has been said, "The truth shall set you free, but first it will tick you off." I shall always remain especially grateful to three persons, one of them then a child, who with just a few words illuminated paths for me that I follow to this day. It is with everlasting appreciation to them for teaching without intending or knowing their impact on me that I share these stories.

I recall one morning in 1950 with special poignancy. I had volunteered to see that our son, then about seven years old, was properly breakfasted and ready for school on time. Still in my impatient mode and eager to get to work, I repeatedly found David only partially dressed, in reverie, or absorbed in a favorite book or in some other diversion. After several increasingly angry commands from me to "step on it," David said, "You know, Daddy, you get mad too easy. You ought to save it for something important."

The humiliating impact of that innocent remark (I silently wished that I could sink through the floor) was such that I cannot recall my response, but I do know that I hurt for several days afterward. I began, however, with increasing effectiveness to ask myself as I felt anger rising, "Wait. Is this important?" By using that device, I found that I could defuse the threatening explosion and even laugh inwardly at the absurd disproportion between the aborted explosion and the stimulus that triggered it. I see this now as an important turning point in my life.

The second incident occurred, as I recall, a year or two later. This was still when I was continually frustrated by colleagues who, I felt at the time, stubbornly refused to appreciate the beauty of my vision, the obvious soundness of my proposals regarding college policies and programs, and the irrefutable logic of my supporting arguments. When I learned that a new friend, Lawrence K. Frank, author of several books on human behavior and interpersonal relationships, was scheduled to lecture at a neighboring university, I persuaded him to visit me at the medical college to see for himself the impasse I had described to him. During his two-day visit, he sat patiently and silently through meetings of various faculty committees and councils of which I was then a member or chairman. After the last of the meetings, we stopped for lunch on the way to the airport for his return flight.

"Well, Larry," I asked, "do you now see what I have to deal with?"

"But, Kim," he responded, "you don't give people any bridges!"

That simple truth immediately penetrated with the sharp, lasting pain of self-disclosure. Larry's observation was right on target. I expected not only my colleagues, but also my family and friends, to always see the rightness of my position and to come to it regardless of where they stood and the directions in which they faced. I learned eventually not so much to give bridges or even to meet others halfway, but to go to where they stood and see what was to be seen from their points of view. I often found it no less valid than what I saw from mine. As the adversarial tensions created by my unyielding self-righteousness eased, more and more of my associates found themselves willing to come and have a look at things from my now more enlightened and accessible viewpoint. With rapprochement came a sharing of goals and more rapid progress toward them. I eventually became aware that living in anger at intransigent colleagues who were part of my daily environment was as stupid and self-defeating as ranting at the weather. I came to love my colleagues as good friends.

The third incident occurred at some forgotten interval after the "bridge" one. A physician trustee of the Kirksville College of Osteopathic Medicine whom I regarded with affectionate esteem repeatedly urged me to accept an assignment on behalf of the college for which he felt I was peculiarly well suited and which would be of great value to the college. Not feeling qualified or interested, I politely declined each time. One evening at an annual college celebration, the doctor's wife, who was also a good friend, sought me out, confided her husband's disappointment, and asked why I would not take on the project even though, as I acknowledged, it would enormously benefit the college. My answer was immediate and emphatic: "Because I can't!"

Her response was as quick but much gentler than mine. "Kim, have you ever thought of saying, 'I haven't been able to' instead of 'I can't'?"

Though softly spoken, that question blew open doors that I had not known were closed to me. I learned that I had been, and needn't continue to be, imprisoned in my own past. Though present and future are undeniably shaped by what has gone before, what has gone before need not set limits on what follows. After all, isn't one measure of progress the limitations that we break through? I accepted the trustee's challenge and found that, while I wasn't at the time able, I did with persistence become able and did produce the anticipated results. I have learned from the experience of the past few decades that, whatever the arena, the acceptance of challenges beyond one's existing abilities prepares one to meet them.

IMPRISONMENT BEHIND NONEXISTENT WALLS

As I wrote about these door openings and breakthroughs, I was reminded of another much more recent incident that gives emphasis to the meaning of "I can't" versus "I haven't been able to." In the fall of 1985, I was a member of a delegation of physicians and scientists invited to China to engage in scientific exchanges with Chinese physicians. In each city, we were taken to our hotel in a special bus, after which we again boarded the bus for a tour of the city.

In Shanghai, the young woman who was our tour guide announced that we would first visit "Old Town, the original walled city." After a short drive, she signaled the driver to stop and informed us that we were within the walls of Old Town. Looking around and finding none, we asked, "Where are the walls?"

The question seemed to startle her. "Oh," she said, "they have been gone for hundreds of years!"

This is, I feel, a perfect metaphor for the perceived but nonexistent walls within which we live our lives, walls that are erected for us by our parents, our teachers, our media, our churches, our cultures, and ourselves. Too few of us wander out to the walls to test their penetrability, being content to live circumscribed lives in accordance with prescribed ways of perceiving, believing, thinking, and behaving. Even fewer of us shake off our culturally induced consensus trance to walk through the walls into a freer, richer, healthier, expanded, and more fulfilling life. Though most of us become well adjusted to the myths, to the nonexistent walls, and to the colored glasses of our culture, can one be said to be well adjusted when the adaptation is to teachings and learnings that American writer and humorist Josh Billings said "ain't so"?[2]

CONTROL, CHALLENGE, COMMITMENT

Not until I came upon the research of psychologists Suzanne Kobasa and Salvatore Maddi and their colleagues did I begin to understand that improvements in health and well-being were a natural and predictable consequence when healthy cognitive structures or ways of viewing reality were available as a method of adaptation to stress.[3] This reminds us that principle II, structure function, applies not only to the musculoskeletal system (or body armor) but also to mental structures. (Remember the flexibility in behavior that followed my newly found physical flexibility.) In addition, their work supports principle IV, meaning drives expectancy, as you will understand when I describe their findings.

In a series of studies on groups of people who, because of shared situations or vocations, were subject to similar severe and chronic stress, Kobasa and Maddi departed from the conventional approach. Instead of limiting themselves to studying the ways some members of each group became ill, they sought to find out what there was about the hardy ones in each group who remained well and who thrived in the face of the same and or even more severe stresses. Two hundred executives of the Illinois Bell Telephone Company who had experienced especially severe and numerous stresses during the AT&T divestiture were evaluated by Kobasa and Maddi's research team. Half suffered severe symptoms and illness, while the others remained essentially symptom free. The evaluation results found that the symptom-free or hardy group had a more successful and effective way of looking at and dealing with all the stressful events and circumstances than did those who succumbed. The one hundred hardy ones viewed changes and problems, such as those that confronted them, as inevitable aspects of life and even as challenging opportunities for personal and professional growth rather than as threats to security and survival. They had somehow acquired a sense of control, namely, control over the psychological and physiological impact of the situation, if not of the situation itself.

This group also manifested high levels of commitment to life, their work, their families, and their own well-being, which subsequently imparted a strong sense of purpose, direction, and enthusiasm.

In their studies of members of other professions and groups, Kobasa and her coworkers found again that one's beliefs, values, attitudes, and learned responses far outweigh the stressor itself in determining its impact on health and well-being. According to Kobasa and her collaborators, the three Cs, defined by strong senses of control, challenge, and commitment, mostly characterize the hardy, stress- and illness-resistant person. The hardy ones seem to have learned, as Hans Selye phrased it, to deal with stress without distress.[4]

On the basis of his own studies, epidemiologist and physician Leonard A. Sagan has independently come to similar conclusions.[5] He offers a list of eight interrelated characteristics common to healthy, stress-resistant people. The eight traits, at least by implication, seem to be elaborations of the senses of control, challenge, and commitment. He sees the hardy people as:

1. Having a high level of self-esteem, possessing an inner locus of control, and believing that what they do and think will matter;
2. Being committed to goals other than their own personal welfare;
3. Placing high values on health and survival;
4. Being oriented to the future, with a willingness to delay immediate gratification for future gain;
5. Trusting in others and being able to form strong and affectionate bonds with others;
6. While relishing companionship, enjoying solitude and opportunities for quiet contemplation and reflection;
7. Pursuing knowledge of themselves, others, and the world around them; and
8. Having a high sense of coherence and confidence that things will work out.

These mental structures seem to support healthy function and interact with the bodymind to maintain health.

THE MATTER OF CHOICE

In commenting on the Kobasa-Maddi studies, psychologist Blair Justice states, "The psychological hardiness studies helped to confirm a basic proposition: The sense of control that is crucial to coping effectively and staying healthy is largely a belief, which we can either adopt or reject. How aversive or damaging an event is depends on how we choose to take it—which means that we can control its effects on our bodies and health by our attitudes and beliefs. Acquiring a sense of control can thus come from recognizing that we can have a powerful impact on our bodily processes by what we do in our heads."[6]

I would like to add my emphasis to what I regard as the key word in this quotation. The impact of an event, a change, a situation, or a problem depends to a crucial degree "on how we *choose* to take it": this is an important example of the options open to humans that are not available to other species. Clearly, the response of the person is a stronger determinant of the effect of stress than the nature, duration, or intensity of the stressor. It is not the stress that kills, another unnecessarily victimizing belief common in our society, but the individual response that kills. That response, in turn, is determined by one's mental structures or mind-set. Once rigid structures are freed up, one can become aware of nonproductive attitudes and knee-jerk responses, and one's mind-set can be changed if one chooses, as I did.

SOCIAL SUPPORT

Complementing the personal health-supporting factors emphasized by Kobasa and her group, by Sagan, and by others are many authors, mainly sociologists and epidemiologists, who have emphasized social factors. Their findings strongly reinforce the conclusion that social support, the sense of belonging and affiliation, and sharing with others an adherence to a set of beliefs, principles, goals, or dedication to a cause are important contributors to health as reflected in a relative freedom from illness, in coping ability, and in longevity. Having a place or a role in one's community as well as opportunities for interaction in a larger social structure has also been shown to engender positive health factors. Other studies have shown that married men have more competent immune systems and longer lives than unmarried men and that those who form close friendships also have health records superior to those who do not. Reviews of these studies can be found in books by Justice, Pelletier, and Pilisuk and Parks as well as in a 1990 issue of the journal *Advances*.[7]

I have been fortunate in these respects, also, as illustrated by the experiences of my second forty-year period. As I said in chapter 1, I came to the Kirksville College of Osteopathic Medicine in 1945 at the age of thirty-six, uncertain that I had made the right decision, despite the strong recommendations of distinguished scientists whose opinions I valued and who had firsthand knowledge of the institution. I soon found myself challenged, however, by the new and fascinating theoretical questions raised in my mind by my early exposure to new (to me) perspectives of health and disease. I became committed to the pursuit of the answers and to the teaching of physiology in the context of the uniqueness of the human species and the differences among humans.

From the first of my many published reports in my new research arena, the osteopathic medical profession has been generous in its expression of appreciation for my contributions to the understanding of underlying biological mechanisms and for my interpretations of the clinical implications of the research findings. In 1979, in celebration of my seventieth birthday, a volume of my collected papers was produced, prefaced by several thoughtful assessments of my work.[8] An additional volume, in commemoration of fifty years of association with the osteopathic medical profession, was published in 1997.[9]

Once they forgave me for my exacting standards, some of the physicians who were once in my classes have also been generous in their acknowledgments of the insights into human physiology to which I led them. Many eventually became fellow faculty members and friends. I have, through the years, served two college presidents and several deans and department heads who once sat in my classes. In my most recent faculty position, three of my former students were my bosses—the college president, a dean, and my department head. Still another student was the coordinator of an interdisciplinary course in which I participated. In short, I am blessed by a large support group and many friends. I have no doubt that they have been important factors in my good health.

So as my understanding of the new medical philosophy deepened, the implications of that philosophy to the practice of medicine in general and to personal and public health became clearer in my mind. I found myself, as a teacher, author, and researcher, increasingly dedicated to the promotion of medical reform.

As is discussed in appendix 1, the spectacular technological advances in medicine do not obviate the need for medical reform, and the problems attending those advances make reform all the more urgent. It is becoming more widely appreciated that the needed reform is not only in the organization, distribution, and economics of healthcare, but also in its basic goals and strategies. The pervasive sense of being a part of such a movement, presently gathering momentum, has also filled my life with purpose, excitement, and fulfillment (principle IV). I have no doubt that this has contributed significantly to the competence of my internal healthcare jester. I think the same can be said of the fact that I have been married—both loved and loving—most of my adult life.

While, as I have said, I have been extraordinarily fortunate with respect to social support and the sense of belonging and of appreciation, virtually all of us, if we are willing to seek and to acknowledge, have had such rewards and have had access to more through our jobs, volunteer services, organizations, places of worship, families, roles in communities, and contributions to the pleasure and welfare of others. Among my happiest experiences in my own volunteer work with groups of older people has been in witnessing the revitalization of those who, on recovering some degree of mobility, come out of inactive retirement to volunteer their diverse services to others in the community and to become activists in causes that are important to them.

OTHER FACTORS IN MY GOOD FORTUNE

In the early 1980s, I discovered and read with great interest *The Relaxation Response* by Herbert Benson, MD, a professor at Harvard Medical School.[10] After practicing the meditation described in the book for two or three years, I was moved to take instruction in transcendental meditation, which I practiced faithfully until 1993. Seated comfortably with my eyes closed in a quiet room each morning and evening, I sought to clear my mind of all thoughts while focusing on my breathing and the silent saying of my mantra. The effect, I discovered, was one of internal quietude and relaxation, which nevertheless prepared me for activity with a minimum of energy-wasting stress. I was most aware of the effect during my daily rush-hour drives on city expressways between home and work. Although I remained alert in heavy traffic, I found myself emotionally untaxed by the behavior of other drivers, congestion, noise, and sluggish traffic lights.

After moving to Boulder, Colorado, I was offered the opportunity to participate as a volunteer in the gerontology program at Naropa Institute, where I heard for the first time about Shambhala meditation. In 1993, I enrolled in a series of intensive weekend training sessions on the underlying philosophy and the "sitting practice" of Shambhala meditation, which I intend to continue for the rest of my life.

For this meditation, I sit upon a small pillow placed on the floor with my legs crossed in front of me and my body erect in an alert posture. My eyes are open as I concentrate on my breath. Stray thoughts, whether about mundane trivia or precious new insights into old problems, are silently acknowledged as *thinking*, an unavoidable aspect of human nature. Without judgment of self or of the thought, I return to concentrating on each phase of each breath. I treasure not only the "at easiness" of this meditation but especially the mindfulness and the deep sense of presence in the here and now. I welcome the less and less frequent judgment of self and others that has come with my Shambhala meditation.

As I continue my daily meditation, I have observed that while I may be aware of anticipatory tension before an important speaking engagement, a committee meeting about a controversial and deeply felt issue, or some other challenge, there is less and less of the futile, adversarial, intrusive, and self-impairing stress. Readers might find books by Chögyam Trungpa, Jon Kabat-Zinn, and Jack Kornfield on this and related subjects inspiring and instructive.[11]

There are, of course, nonmeditative techniques for bringing about one's own more positive behaviors, feelings, and responses and for the accompanying functional improvements in the immune and other systems. These include self-hypnosis, autogenic training, imagery, and biofeedback. You will find these described and evaluated in books by Justice, Borysenko, Rossman, Pelletier, Achterberg, and others previously cited in this chapter and others.

BODY AWARENESS

Although I have had no training in biofeedback, through the years I have acquired sufficient body awareness to quickly detect muscular or other bodily tension and postural changes that reflect even slight uneasiness. I can then do something about it either by addressing the source of the uneasiness, when I can identify it, or by the physical manifestation of it. Often the physical manifestation and the psychological discomfort can be eliminated by a small change in posture, such as dropping my shoulders, a change in facial expression, or by a moment's focus on my breathing. The physical expression of the psychological discomfort, I have found, actually exacerbates and sustains the psychological discomfort. Conversely, elimination of the physical signs often breaks the vicious circle and is another example of principle I, interactive unity.

I had a striking and totally unexpected demonstration of this phenomenon several years ago on one of my morning runs. As I started out, I was aware that I was not feeling my best. Around the usual midway point, I felt myself approaching utter exhaustion. I was about to interrupt the run and slowly walk the rest of the way home when I became aware that my face was contorted in a jaw-clenched grimace that expressed all-out effort and strain such as is often seen on the faces of runners as they cross the finish line in a race. I remember calling for repose and then feeling the muscles of my head and face relax and let go. Fueled by a parallel release of available energy, I sailed home.

I have the same experience when walking or driving into the bright sun. The reflexive response to this unpleasant stimulus seems to call on the facial musculature to narrow the space between the eyelids that usually produces an expression that signals the discomfort. By conscious attention, I have learned how to lower the upper lids without evoking the grimace of distress and thereby eliminating the distress itself.

You may be wondering why I have chosen to describe so many personal experiences; I have reviewed them to illustrate some advantages of learning how to observe and listen to one's body for clues to one's mental and emotional state and to its improvement. I also wanted to broaden the application of structure function iterated in principle II to include the structures of the mind and the spirit; to offer additional illustrations of the interactive unity of the mind, body, and spirit discussed in principle I; and to point out the self-healing that occurs when a structure is improved as described in principle III. In addition, I wanted to offer illustrations of the importance of meaning and expectancy that compose principle IV and to illustrate how the utilization of the new brain (neocortex) aids in transcending difficult circumstances through control, challenge, and commitment.

Finally, I would like to remind you that quality of life includes enjoyment of life, work, personal relationships, and leisure. It even includes enjoyment of stress and discipline! As Norman Cousins has so dramatically demonstrated, fun and laughter have a powerful positive influence on the bodymind's own healthcare system.[12] In the circular manner that characterizes life's processes and in contrast to the linear cause-and-effect manner usually ascribed to inanimate phenomena, I believe joy, fun, and laughter favor the maintenance, restoration, and enhancement of health, just as good health enhances the capacity for joy, fun, and laughter. I, for one, am grateful for my own sense of humor and for the pleasure it gives to others.

This chapter on changing the mind has been dedicated (1) to identifying behavioral, attitudinal, and psychosocial factors that contribute to the enhancement of personal potential and well-being in all aspects of one's life and (2) to demonstrating that, if one chooses, it is possible even late in life to replace maladaptive, self-defeating, unnecessarily stressful, and health-impairing behaviors with others that feel good and are self-empowering, gratifying, health enhancing, and life preserving.

In the next and final chapter, I have tried to draw together all of the foregoing lessons that I learned during my second forty-year life about health, its sources, and its ups and downs. I also intend to highlight those lessons that are most relevant to aging successfully and to "dying young when you're very old."

NOTES

1. T. H. Holmes and R. H. Rahe, "The Social Readjustment Rating Scale," *Journal of Psychosomatic Research* 11 (1967): 213–18.

2. J. Billings, *Josh Billings, Hiz Sayings* (Kila, MT: Kessinger, 2006).

3. S. C. Kobasa, "Commitment and Coping in Stress Resistance among Lawyers," *Journal of Personality and Social Psychology* 42 (1982): 707–17; S. C. Kobasa, S. R. Maddi, and S. Courington, "Personality and Constitution as Mediators in the Stress-Illness Relationship," *Journal of Health and Social Behavior* 22 (1981): 368–78; S. C. Kobasa, S. R. Maddi, and S. Kahn, "Hardiness and Health: A Prospective Study," *Journal of Personality and Social Psychology* 42 (1982): 168–77; S. R. Maddi and S. C. Kobasa, *The Hardy Executive: Health under Stress* (Homewood, IL: Dow Jones-Irwin, 1984).

4. H. Selye, *The Stress of Life* (New York: McGraw-Hill, 1976).

5. L. A. Sagan, *The Health of Nations* (New York: Basic Books, 1987).

6. B. Justice, *Who Gets Sick: Thinking and Health* (Houston: Peak Press, 1987).

7. Ibid.; K. R. Pelletier, *Mind as Healer, Mind as Slayer: A Holistic Approach to Preventing Stress Disorders* (New York: Delta, 1977); M. Pilisuk and S. H. Parks, *The Healing Web: Social Networks and Human Survival* (Boston: University Press of New England, 1986); H. F. Andrews, "Helping and Health: The Relationship between Volunteer Activity and Health-Related Outcomes," *Advances* 7 (1990): 25–34; S. Cohen, "Social Support and Physical Illnesses," *Advances* 7 (1990): 35–47.

8. B. Peterson, ed., *The Collected Papers of Irvin M. Korr* (Colorado Springs, CO: American Academy of Osteopathy, 1979).

9. H. H. King, ed., *The Collected Papers of Irvin M. Korr*, vol. 2 (Indianapolis: American Academy of Osteopathy, 1997).

10. H. Benson and M. Z. Klipper, *The Relaxation Response* (New York: Avon, 1976).

11. C. Trungpa, *Shambhala: The Sacred Path of the Warrior* (Boston: Shambhala, 1988); J. Kabat-Zinn, *Wherever You Go, There You Are* (New York: Hyperion, 1994); J. Kabat-Zinn, *Coming to Our Senses* (New York: Hyperion, 2005); J. Kornfield, *A Path with Heart* (New York: Bantam, 1993).

12. N. Cousins, *Anatomy of an Illness as Perceived by the Patient* (New York: Norton, 1979).

PART 5

REINFORCEMENT OF LESSONS LEARNED

"Having lived according to the laws of nature, I can expect to die young—when I am very old."

—I. M. Korr

Chapter 16

THE LAST OF LIFE FOR WHICH THE FIRST WAS MADE

Usual or Successful Aging, Your Choice

"The less distinct the boundary between me and the rest of the universe, the more distinct is my identity."

—I. M. Korr

THE HEALTH OF AN AGING POPULATION

Appendix 1 explains in some detail a paradoxical national problem: the lower the morbidity (the incidence of disease in the population), the lower the mortality; but the lower the mortality, the higher the morbidity. This paradox is very pertinent because of the enormous burden of chronic illness that continues to grow as more and more people live into their later decades. In addition, this paradox remains true despite the fact that the average level of health among the elderly has improved and has further increased our life expectancy. The problem will continue to grow, certainly well into the twenty-first century, and at an immense and perhaps insupportable cost to the nation's economy. Therefore, this problem must be addressed as assiduously at its roots with health promotion as it has been addressed at its terminal branches through disease treatment.

Chronic illness will continue to afflict larger numbers of older persons as long as medical policies and practices, as well as the medical education and training for those who are responsible for the policies and practices, continue to be guided by the premise that chronic degenerative diseases are a natural, intrinsic, and inescapable aspect of aging. Based on that premise, it follows that any major investment in prevention is inadvisable because it would divert precious resources from the many who are already afflicted, thus further darkening the gloomy picture.

At present, most (about 96 percent) of the nation's health bill goes for after-the-fact palliative treatment of existing, advanced, and terminal disease and for prolonging the last year or two of life. Only the remaining 4 percent, approximately, goes toward prevention, such as early detection and treatment of existing disease (for example, breast cancer), and for such public health measures as immunization of children.[1] And only a fraction of that goes for the promotion of health, even though it is the most comprehensive, effective, and economical form of disease prevention. While the underlying premise of this book has been that the higher the level of health, the lower the probability of disease, whatever the age, currently our health resources are focused on disease treatment rather than health promotion.

As Dr. Anne Somers and J. M. McGinnis point out, the gloomy statistics demonstrate not the inadvisability but the urgency of expanding the nation's investment in prevention.[2] Increased support of such agencies of the Public Health Service as the Office of Disease Prevention and Health Promotion and the Centers for Disease Control and Prevention, as well as the implementation of the national health agenda set forth in 1979, 1980, 2000, and 2010 is vital.[3] In fact, government initiatives have made some progress in decreasing heart disease, and serious efforts are given to obesity and smoking cessation.[4]

However, even these excellent programs and proposals fail to draw a fundamental distinction that was enunciated in part by the World Health Organization as long ago as 1947[5] and which is the pervasive theme of this book; that distinction is between high-level health and well-being on the one hand and merely low morbidity (the absence of disease and infirmity) on the other. Nor is there significant appreciation of the fact that while attention to risk factors alone may improve the morbidity statistics, it does not by itself produce high-level health. Still, the higher the level of health, the better the morbidity statistics.

That last point was unintentionally dramatized in the findings of the Stanford Heart Disease Prevention Program directed by John W. Farquhar, MD.[6] This is, I think, my favorite how-to book on health promotion even though, in the prevailing mode, it is primarily addressed to preventing a specific disease. In the introduction, Farquhar places responsibility for health squarely on the shoulders of the individual, saying that nobody else can assume that responsibility, "not the doctor, not a fleet of doctors. In the way we live our lives, we either enhance our health or diminish it." He then describes, briefly and simply, with ample latitude for individual taste, health status, and abilities, what makes up a healthy lifestyle. It is refreshingly different from the glut of health books that promise quick and easy gimmicks for curing or preventing everything from wrinkles to cancer. Although published in 1978, it deals with enduring principles that remain unaltered by today's or even tomorrow's breakthroughs. The prevention program he provides includes such components as certain behavioral and psychological adjustments, exercise, dietary changes, weight control, and, of course, smoking cessation. What emerges, apparently unexpectedly, is that the healthful changes in lifestyle prevent (that is, substantially lower the incidence of) not only heart disease but other serious diseases as well.

Therefore, what is required is a much better balance between the preventive approach, which gets to the roots of the problem, and the remedial approach, which gets to the terminal branches. By roots, I mean those life paths or ways of living that, with the passing of time, naturally culminate in one or more of the long-term diseases and infirmities that lower the quality of life and burden our society. By the preventive approach, I mean moving the tens of millions of people not yet sick, who are the vast reservoir in which the diseases originate (and of which I was a part until my forties), to paths, such as my present one, that culminate in a healthy old age.

INDIVIDUAL HEALTH IN AN AGING POPULATION: THE LESSONS TO BE LEARNED

How do national health and the tens of millions not yet ill relate to individual health? What is their relation to your health and to your prospects of achieving healthy old age, whether you are still young or very old? Until a much better balance is struck between the therapeutic and preventive approaches, you and as many others as possible (sick or not yet sick, young or old) must be motivated, educated, and enabled to assume responsibility for your own and your family's healthcare while continuing, as necessary, to call on healthcare providers for what they do best—disease care.

As stated in the introduction, this book is intended to enhance your motivation by offering you a more positive perspective about health and the lifetime rewards brought by the steady progression toward the brighter hues on the health spectrum, especially in the later part of life "for which the first was made," to once again quote nineteenth-century British poet Robert Browning.[7]

In continuing that effort in this final chapter, I once again refer to human diversity and, by implication, your uniqueness as a person. The heterogeneity of human life is such that, from the moment of conception, we begin to travel our individual, absolutely unique biological paths. The longer we live, the more our paths diverge and the more heterogeneous we become. Some of us are very old at sixty, some very young; some not yet old at ninety, most dead before ninety. Those old in years cannot be stereotyped, because they are the ultimate in diversity.

What are the lessons to be learned from those who are very young at sixty and those who are not yet old at ninety?

The first question that arose in my mind as I began thinking about this summation was if I were called on to select from all the principles that have guided my life in the past forty or so years, what would be the one that has been the *sine qua non* of my own excellent health at this stage of my life? My choice was immediate and reaffirmed again and again with further thought. It is my appreciation of and confidence in my own indwelling healthcare system that comprises all the body-mind's regulatory, protective, healing, regenerative, compensatory, and recuperative mechanisms. This is my choice because it has led to the acceptance of my lifelong responsibility for the care of that system. As a result, my long commitment to its care, essentially that of doing it a minimum of harm, has been richly rewarded.

As a physiologist with some grasp of the immense complexity of the internal healthcare system; of its numerous, individually complex component systems; and of their functional integration, I remain awed by its utter dependability and competence and by the medical miracles it routinely performs when it is permitted to operate unimpeded by human neglect and abuse. I am convinced that the millions of other men and women who have also lived long, active lives did so as well, even without awareness of their personal healthcare systems, by living in such a way as to sustain and enhance its competence, however personally or genetically determined.

Does this mean that we, the millions of fortunate old men and women, are (or were) invulnerable, free of infirmities, disabilities, or diseases? Not at all. Health promotion, like almost everything else in life, comes without a warranty. Total absence of disease is not guaranteed. What high levels of health do ensure, however, is that illness will be less probable and less severe and that the factors beyond our personal control, such as the genes that happened to pair up at our conception, the pollutants that happened to be injected into the air we breathe as well as the water and food we ingest, and all the traumas and other accidents of life, will be less deleterious. Simply, the risk factors will be less risky. Our illnesses, when they come, are less intrusive in our lives, both in duration and in quality.

I have remained well and active despite chronic diseases, as is true of many others as old or older than I. I am hypertensive, a family trait inherited from the maternal side of my family. My mother was hypertensive, as were her mother and her brother and as is one of my two siblings.

Another problem I have, of unknown origin, is a severe retinopathy (retinal exudative telangiectasia), a noninflammatory disorder of the retina. Vision in my left eye can be corrected by lenses only to 20/200, the right eye to 20/30 or 20/40. I have long made it a practice to carry a pocket flashlight and a magnifying lens to read menus and theater or concert programs in light that is ordinarily quite adequate for others. Despite this condition, I can drive a car, hit and catch a ball, and play tennis competently.

A third problem came to light in 1979 as I prepared, somewhat apprehensively, for a lecture trip to Australia and New Zealand. A severe and painful attack of gout required emergency treatment to enable me to depart on time. This apparent defect in my metabolism is kept under control by my diet and other aspects of my lifestyle.

The second question that came to mind as I pondered over the summation was what motivated me in my early forties to make and keep the commitment as I did, a commitment that made possible an old age that is the best time of my life despite chronic impairments. As I reported early in the book, it was the new feelings that followed the improvement in bodily flexibility, such as my newfound joy of moving and breathing with ease, the freedom from pain, and the new reserves of energy no longer wasted in overcoming friction. Having maintained that flexibility, I still move with the ease, fluidity, and, I am told, grace if not the speed and endurance of a much younger person.

The new mobility and energy enabled me in my early forties to begin to seek and delight in new challenges in personal, professional, and societal realms. Flexibility of body quite naturally, because of the oneness of bodymind, brought with it a belated and all the more welcome openness and flexibility of mind and behavior. The dropping away of my bodymind's too solid armor freely let in, for the first time, the love of others. I also became exposed to self-examination that facilitated further liberating, healthful changes in feelings, attitudes, responses, relationships, and activities. This long and continuing series of changes, initiated by restoration and maintenance of youthful flexibility, has brought me enormous rewards as a researcher, teacher, coworker, friend, husband, and father and as a caring, responsible citizen.

These changes have made it possible for me to continue to be creatively and enthusiastically involved in diverse and challenging activities. Although I look forward to being an active nonagenarian, I accept with equanimity the death that comes closer with each passing day, as it does for us all.

I seem to have but one regret: that, through nobody's fault, I was denied an earlier start on the path I have followed in the second forty-plus period of my life. I find that I can assuage that regret by doing what I can to motivate others, young and old, to make their commitments to health as soon as possible. No year is either too early or too late to start, but the earlier, the better. Indeed, one challenge I look forward to is that of developing, with others, a model program in primary and secondary education in which children can learn and accept responsibility for their own health as one of their future adult responsibilities to society.

As I explained much earlier, I chose to write at length about myself not because my health story is unique or unusual but because my intimate familiarity with that story, when reviewed from my viewpoint as a veteran physiologist and medical educator, led me to insights that have been helpful to other aged adults with whom I have shared them. Countless others are or were far better models of successful aging than I. Unfortunately, they seldom write about *their* health secrets.

MODELS OF SUCCESSFUL AGING

When I consider other models of successful aging, many distinguished names come to mind from diverse areas of endeavor and backgrounds:

Pablo Casals, Pablo Picasso, Leopold Stokowski, George Abbott, Grandma Moses, Martha Graham, Bob Hope, George Bernard Shaw, George Burns, Georgia O'Keeffe, Cab Calloway, Karl A. Menninger, Maggie Kuhn, Linus Pauling, Helen Hayes, Benjamin Spock, Claude Pepper, Lionel Hampton, Justices Marshall and Brennan, Katherine Dunham, Katharine Hepburn, Ella Fitzgerald, Armand Hammer, and Bertrand Russell. Each of us can name others whom we especially admire, famous or not, who have achieved enriched and enriching old age. Sometimes this has been achieved despite chronic disease but always with boundless dedication and enthusiasm.

I select two names from the above list for special comment because of the public attention given to them and because they illustrate so well the importance of continued acceptance of challenges in advanced age, even in the face of serious chronic illness.

Maggie Kuhn was the cofounder and dynamic leader of the national organization of older adults known as the Gray Panthers. She was interviewed in 1990 as part of the celebration of the twentieth anniversary of its founding and of her eighty-fifth birthday.[8] One question was, "Why do you think you have been so successful as the leader of the Gray Panthers?"

Her response was, "In all of the jobs I've ever had, I've always had a goal. Every year I've thought of a new goal to drive me ahead. I love living this way. And it has not always been a piece of cake. I've been ill; I've had cancer three times. I've had many disappointments—there's been sadness and tremendous frustration at points—but my goals lift me and buoy me up. I've had to deal with many changes in my own physical condition—the arthritic pain, vision loss—but the characteristic of my old age is that I've never given up hope; it springs eternal."

Ms. Kuhn died in April 1995 at the age of ninety.

Karl A. Menninger, MD, of the famous Menninger Foundation, distinguished psychiatrist and author of many books and articles, was interviewed on National Public Radio in July 1990, a few days before his ninety-seventh birthday. He was still very much involved in professional affairs, and though his voice was not strong, he was still able to convey his clarity and passion about various public issues (especially about the subject of one of his books, the "crime of punishment"), despite having suffered from strokes and cancer. Dr. Menninger died soon after that interview.

I found many admirable models of successful aging in Fort Worth, Texas, my home from 1978 to 1991. I was part of an organization, the Senior Citizen Alliance, which consisted of about two hundred members whose monthly meetings I often attended as guest and as speaker. The members of the Senior Citizen Alliance are men and women in their sixties, seventies, and eighties, retired from diverse vocations, businesses, and professions, who are representatives of local chapters of the American Association of Retired Persons as well as organizations of retired teachers, federal employees, and others. All are activists, enthusiastically and effectively absorbed in various community projects and volunteer activities that serve others less fortunate than they, from premature infants to nursing home residents and the disabled. They actively participate in Meals on Wheels, in politics as lobbyists (in the Senior PAC and the Silver-Haired Legislature), in legal and financial counseling, as well as in numerous other services, causes, and programs. Many carry on with utter dedication despite disabilities and chronic illnesses.

I have detailed knowledge of the health-related habits of only a few members, but since every meeting begins with a cafeteria luncheon of individually selected food, I was able to observe that most members recognize the importance of healthful diets. Even moderate obesity is most exceptional among them, as are signs of osteoporotic spines, even in the aged women. Indeed, their postures on the whole are exemplary, and, as they carry their trays to tables, they move with ease and with none of the shuffling so common among the elderly. In the discussions and debates that are part of each meeting, their voices are strong and their thinking is clear on diverse issues. I found it a great joy to be among them and to feel their vitality, their good humor, their commitment and enthusiasm, and their power.

Since leaving Fort Worth in September 1991 and reluctantly

parting from my fellow oldsters, I have been delighted to join and to be inspired by their many counterparts in Boulder and neighboring communities in Colorado. I shall never forget how astounded I was as I took my first tentative strides on the ski trails of Eldora to see men and women even older than I skiing not only on the cross-country trails but on the steep downhill slopes, with confidence, speed, and grace.

A few pages back, I referred to the aged persons each of us knows, famous or not, who achieved enriched and enriching old age, often in spite of chronic disease. We also know others who, even though free of disabling infirmities and possessing valuable skills, begin an empty existence upon retirement. When I suggested a few weekly hours of volunteer service to such an acquaintance, he firmly declined, saying, "I've paid my dues." He is by no means alone. I cannot help but feel deeply saddened on my occasional visits to retirement communities when I observe the degree to which so many people, including those who are able and skilled in many fields, are content to devote tens of thousands of man-and-woman years to killing time while they wait to die, as if that is their reward for having paid their dues.

THE CHOICE: USUAL OR SUCCESSFUL AGING

Walter M. Bortz II, MD, prominent geriatrician, has much to say on this very point. "The essence of geriatric medicine," he states, "is found not in disease diagnosis, but in functional capability." He continues, "the medical model needs rethinking and reforming as it confronts the needs of older persons; it needs to emphasize preventive strategies and functional assessment and therapy. Cure becomes secondary to maintenance of maximum vigor and independence. Self-efficacy should become a new gold standard for the third age."[9] (The first two ages are growth and adulthood.)

It would be absurd to deny that there are not normal age-related functional declines or that they do not begin long before the age of sixty-five. We need only look at the early ages at which even the most talented athletes retire and the regularity with which top-seeded tennis players in their early thirties, despite excellent health and fitness, are displaced by teenagers. We can also marvel that Texas Rangers pitcher Nolan Ryan could win his three hundredth game at the advanced age of forty-three. It is to say, however, and as documented in earlier chapters, that much, even most, of the decline in old age—in mobility, physical and mental abilities, competence of body systems, autonomy, interests, loving relationships, pleasure, social activity, and self-esteem—is avoidable because its origin is extrinsic to and superimposed on the intrinsic aging process.

This conclusion was amply substantiated by a research review published in *Science*, one of the two most widely read scientific journals in the world, by Harvard University geriatrician John W. Rowe, MD, and University of Michigan psychologist Robert L. Kahn, PhD.[10] They drew what I regard as a most lucid and incisive distinction between nondisease and optimal health, between disease prevention and health enhancement, between focus on deficits and losses, and focus on assets and potentials. The distinction is succinctly stated in the title of their frequently quoted article, "Human Aging: Usual and Successful."

Rowe and Kahn showed that a high degree of variability is evident in normal, that is, nondiseased, senior citizens of the same age. In a series of physiological tests, some show considerable losses as compared with the average in their younger counterparts, while others have little or no physiological loss. The latter group, the authors state, could be said to have aged more successfully, at least with respect to physiological functions.

The differences between the usual and the successful can be largely ascribed to differences in constellations of factors subsumed under lifestyle; these differences are evident also in the incidence of risk factors for specific diseases. For example, risk factors for heart disease, such as increases in blood pressure, body weight, and serum cholesterol, which are generally assumed to be age related, are usual in the populations that have customarily been studied. That is, they have been studied in prosperous industrial countries but not in agricultural societies.

Given such cross-cultural and within-group variations, Rowe and Kahn offer the hypothesis that the functional losses and increased risk factors commonly attributed to age "may often be exaggerated and that *factors of diet, exercise, nutrition and the like may have been underesti-mated as potential moderators of the aging process*" (emphasis added). If so, they go on to say, then the prospects are favorable for moderating, avoiding, or even reversing functional losses common in the elderly and for reducing the probability of "adverse health outcomes."

The bulk of the Rowe-Kahn article is a review of the research literature demonstrating the often remarkable degree to which pre-cursors of disease can be reduced or eliminated and to which func-tional capacities, including the cognitive, can be improved in aged populations by the modification of extrinsic factors. These include exercise, diet, training and improvement of emotional states by adjusting psychosocial factors in favor of increased autonomy and control, and improved social support. There can be little doubt that much of the physical and mental decline associated with usual aging is largely preventable, modifiable, and reversible. My own personal history and my observations of others who, even late in life, learned the art of successful aging support that hypothesis.

Because of its preoccupation with prevention of illness and post-ponement of death, what is almost entirely overlooked, even in the prevention-oriented clinical literature and practice, is that even very old age can be a time of joy, excitement, enthusiasm, and fulfillment. It can also be a time for giving pleasure and enlightenment to others. The most important thing that we need to realize is that these things are all possible even in the face of chronic illness and disability.

I hope that it has become compellingly clear to my younger readers (and their parents) that it is never too early to begin the process of successful aging and to my older readers that it is never (well, almost never) too late; old age can be and can become a time for exu-berant well-being. The lesson is simple: Keep moving, keep learning, keep reaching, and keep on doing good.

I hope that this book has, if I may borrow the words of Dr. Anne

Somers, brought you "greater recognition of the fundamental fact that health, like life itself, is a precious gift to be celebrated, cherished and nurtured in accordance with the laws of nature."[11] My purpose has been to help you to understand those laws and, by displaying the rewards, to move you to observe the laws henceforth. I remind you for the last time that you are the owner and custodian of a remarkable and irreplaceable legacy that is the product of millions of years of development and refinement—your own healthcare system. May nature's laws be your guide in its care and may they serve you well.

Whatever your age, I hope that this book has conveyed something helpful to you about the art of healthful living and, as George Burns, centenarian actor-comedian put it, about the art of growing older without getting old. Whether or not you have been able to avoid major illness, we are mortal and destined to die from the failure of some function or other. The ultimate preventive goal of truly successful aging is to compress all illness into the final moments of life.[12]

In the meantime, enjoy, enjoy!

NOTES

1. "US Preventive Medicine Introduces Next Generation of Healthcare in America," US Preventive Medicine, http://www.uspreventivemedicine .com/Press-Room/USPM-News/USPM_Launch.html (accessed March 28, 2007).

2. J. M. McGinnis, "The Tithonus Syndrome: Health and Aging in America," in *Health Promotion and Disease Prevention in the Elderly*, ed. R. Chernoff and D. A. Lipschitz (New York: Raven, 1988), pp. 1–15; A. R. Somers, "Preventive Health Services for the Elderly: The Growing Consensus," in *Health Promotion*, ed. Chernoff and Lipschitz, pp. 17–32.

3. United States Public Health Service, "Healthy People: The Surgeon General's Report on Health Promotion and Disease Prevention," 1979, http:// profiles.nlm.nih.gov/NN/B/B/G/K/ (accessed March 2, 2007); US Public Health Service, *Promoting Health/Preventing Disease: Objectives for the Nation* (Rockville, MD: US Public Health Service, 1980); "Healthy People

2000," US Department of Health and Human Services, http://odphp .osophs.dhhs.gov/PUBS/HP2000/default.htm (accessed March 23, 2007); "Healthy People 2010," US Department of Health and Human Services, http://www.healthypeople.gov/ (accessed March 23, 2007).

4. "Healthy People 2010 Spotlight," National Center for Health Statistics, http://www.cdc.gov/nchs/hphome.htm (accessed March 23, 2007).

5. World Health Organization, "About WHO," 2007, http://www .who.int/about/en/ (accessed February 28, 2007).

6. J. W. Farquhar, *The American Way of Life Need Not Be Hazardous to Your Health* (New York: Norton, 1978).

7. R. Browning, "Rabbi Ben Ezra," in *Robert Browning*, ed. A. Roberts (Oxford: Oxford University Press, 1997), pp. 304–10.

8. A. Lederman, "Interview with Maggie Kuhn," *Gray Panther Network* 19 (1990): 3–5.

9. W. H. Bortz, "Geriatrics: Through the Looking Glass," *Medical Times* (June 1989): 85–92.

10. J. W. Rowe and R. L. Kahn, "Human Aging: Usual and Successful," *Science* 237 (1987): 143–49.

11. Somers, "Preventive Health Services for the Elderly."

12. J. W. Rowe and R. L. Kahn, *Successful Aging* (New York: Pantheon, 1998).

EPILOGUE
Rene J. McGovern, PhD

"First the material body, second the spiritual being, third a being of mind which is far superior to all vital motions and material forms, whose duty is to wisely manage this great engine of life."
—A. T. Still from *Philosophy of Osteopathy*

I n this epilogue, I would like to introduce you very briefly to a history of osteopathic medicine; offer you a glimpse of the work that is being done worldwide to evaluate osteopathic philosophy and practice; and, finally review and help you apply the principles that Dr. Korr embraced and wanted to share with you.

Throughout the centuries, physicians, scientists, philosophers, and thinkers of all kinds have pondered the body's amazing healing ability. Some have sought to go beyond the physical to examine the mental and spiritual aspects of healing. Beginning in 1892, Andrew Taylor Still, MD, DO, the founder of the osteopathic medical profession, wrote numerous papers, articles, and books promoting a revolutionary holistic approach to healthcare.[1] Dr. Still stated in his autobiography that he spent twenty years learning and perfecting osteopathic medicine prior to founding a new type of medical school in Kirksville, Missouri, when he was sixty-five years old.[2] The plan to build this school was strongly encouraged by Kirksville leaders and businessmen who feared that because of his advanced age Dr. Still might die at any time. Initially, Kirksville's citizens were looking out for their own self-interests; the loss of Dr. Still's unique medical skills without trained followers would jeopardize the town's newly gained revenue from the thousands of patients coming from various parts of the country for osteopathic treatments. Unfortunately, they did not really understand "the old doctor" who practiced medicine without relying on the often harmful drugs of the times and who could heal crippled bodies with his hands.[3] Dr. Still lived to be eighty-nine years old.

Today, the osteopathic profession has grown to include more than twenty-six medical schools. The increasing popularity of these schools is attributed to their emphasis on treating the whole person—body, mind, and spirit. The founding school of osteopathic medicine, Kirksville College of Osteopathic Medicine (KCOM), is now part of A. T. Still University (ATSU). In addition to the original goal of training osteopathic physicians, the ATSU system also integrates osteo-pathic principles into the training of other health professions, including physical therapy, occupational therapy, sports medicine, human move-ment, audiology, dentistry, and health management. In addition to the doctoral degree in osteopathic medicine, the university offers doctoral degrees in physical therapy, audiology, health education, health sci-ences, and dentistry. The university now also offers a master's degree in biomedical research and in twelve other areas of healthcare.

Since its founding in 1892, the osteopathic profession has been concerned mainly with healthcare provision and not with research. However, the need for research into the philosophy and practices of osteopathic medicine has existed for many years.[4] Beginning in the mid-1940s and continuing for the next three decades, a large body of data relating to osteopathic medicine was gathered in Kirksville, Mis-souri, by Irvin M. Korr, PhD; J. Stedman Denslow, DO; and others. Drs. Korr and Denslow developed techniques that allowed them to build a strong scientific foundation on which future osteopathic researchers could expand. A compendium of Dr. Korr's work, including that done with Dr. Denslow, has been published in *The Collected Papers of Irvin M. Korr*, volumes 1 and 2.[5] Unfortunately, for years their promising work languished, known only to the few who had developed an interest in studying the concepts of manual medicine embodied in the techniques of osteopathic medicine.

In 1997, when my husband, James J. McGovern, PhD, became the ninth president of the Kirksville College of Osteopathic Medicine, a resurgence of support and an acknowledgment of the importance of osteopathic research occurred. President McGovern recognized the demographic needs of an aging society and, coming from major research universities, foresaw the advent of evidence-based medicine and the application of best practices as setting the standard for medical care in the future.[6] Both of us saw the great potential of osteopathic medicine for fulfilling these future needs and wanted to do what was necessary to strengthen its influence around the world.[7] As he had done at previous institutions, President McGovern provided the necessary leadership and infrastructure for productive research programs. He also became a spokesperson nationally and internationally for the primacy of osteopathic principles to health and the need for evidence of their effectiveness.[8] (Please note that our book *Your Healer Within* has printed versions in English, Spanish, and German.)

Although well suited to meet the demands of an aging society, osteopathy may be limited in its ability to respond to the challenge of evidence-based medicine to demonstrate efficacy.[9] This challenge may arise because of difficulties in applying the gold standard research model of the randomized controlled study (RCT) in the osteopathic medical setting. This concern has been addressed most recently in an editorial in the *Journal of the American Osteopathic Association* written by Michael Patterson, PhD, a former colleague of Dr. Korr's. In discussing the difficulties of research design and, in particular, providing an appropriate sham control for osteopathic manipulative treatment (OMT), Dr. Patterson quotes Dr. Korr's work:

> It is essential . . . that assessments of effectiveness of OMT be of OMT *as it is practiced*, as an integral part of the total interaction between physician and patient, and not as an isolated, contrived, and standardized procedure. . . . The placebo response is an integral, inseparable part of the patient's total response to osteopathic medical care.[10]

Osteopathic researchers worldwide are responding to the challenges of demonstrating the efficacy of osteopathic medicine.[11] Don Noll, DO, FACOI, osteopathic researcher, geriatrician, and professor of internal medicine at A. T. Still University, in a recent article reviewed current clinical research in osteopathy.[12] He noted that promising research has been done on the broad application of osteopathy not only to musculoskeletal problems but also to primarily visceral organ systems, or systemic disorders, such as pneumonia and influenza,[13] and to decreasing the length of stay in hospitals.[14] Research is also being done on the impact on chronic progressive diseases, such as Parkinson's disease.[15] Additional osteopathic studies are looking at the prevention of falls[16] and the decrease in range of motion,[17] problems that are frequently predictors of aging and of the need for assisted care. Through the support of the American Osteopathic Association (AOA), the Heritage Foundation, and the National Center for Complementary and Alternative Medicine (CAM) of the National Institutes of Health (NIH) and through collaborative efforts, such as those through the osteopathic research center in Texas and other collaborations worldwide between MD and DO researchers, osteopathic researchers are becoming more sophisticated in their ability to refine research questions and objectively measure outcomes.[18]

Inherent in the struggle to conduct valid research on osteopathic care, however, is the distinction between a discrete intervention, such as the administration of a particular medication and the evaluation of an approach to care that involves a relationship. Thus, is a "dose" of manipulation, such as Dr. Chace gave Dr. Korr during his first osteopathic treatment, something that can be randomized and controlled?

The "nuisance variable" or placebo response that Dr. Korr referred to in an earlier chapter is part and parcel of that relationship.[19] It is the caring and teaching that helps change one's beliefs and that made Dr. Korr shift from expecting poor health and an early death to spending the next fifty years expecting and enjoying good health. Further, his continuous evaluation and further application of that comprehensive relational approach to care allowed him to share his "secrets" with you.

Underlying the challenges and the historical controversy of osteopathy are, I believe, the very principles that Dr. Korr espoused and wished to impart.[20] As Dr. Korr told us in the introduction of this book, the four principles described in part 2 have been articulated across the centuries. In *Your Healer Within*, my husband and I explained that the four principles align with the four explanations of reality, which were articulated by Aristotle as the formal, the material, the efficient, and the final cause. These are the foundational elements of numerous approaches to living the good life and dying a good death, including those of the major world religions. Sometimes the fine line between the art of the practice of medicine and enthusiasm for a belief system can become blurred. Sometimes, too, the science of medicine can be emphasized to the detriment of the underlying belief system or human context of its application. Dr. Korr was very balanced in his lifetime contributions to both the science and the critical development and artic- ulation of the theoretical framework within which people could under- stand and apply the evidence of these principles in very practical ways. This quality is what makes a great scientist.

The osteopathic principles present a way of life that will enable you to more fully express your individuality, to enjoy life, and to achieve your highest potential. As a health psychologist, I was struck by Dr. Korr's articulation of key concepts that have been supported in psy- chological research on health and well-being. First is the importance of individual choice and the perception of control; next is the importance of social support; finally is the critical need to break through cognitive barriers or the rigid structures that Dr. Korr describes as "crumbling" after his first osteopathic treatment.[21] As you read his chapters, you experience his delight at his metamorphosis from the rigid, type A professor to one who felt love toward his colleagues and new openness toward his students. Repeatedly, right until the end of his life, he revels in seeing reality in new ways. (See p. 193 in chapter 16.) His method of evaluating his experiences and challenging his thoughts is a key process in cognitive behavioral therapy. Cognitive behavioral therapy is a mode of psychological treatment that has the most evidence supporting its efficacy for the treatment of depression, anxiety, and other emotional difficulties that can challenge people in the course of living. In cognitive behavioral therapy, patients are taught about the relationship between thoughts, feelings, and behavior. As they become aware of dysfunctional, rigid thoughts that often drive their behavior and cause uncomfortable feelings, they become better able to replace them with more appropriate thoughts and free themselves from their emotional chains.[22]

Oftentimes, the body is the source of awareness of the thoughts. This knowledge has been incorporated into therapeutic methods that help patients develop both awareness of the body and the thoughts through such techniques as mindfulness meditation.[23] In *Living Long and Loving It*, Dr. Korr repeatedly gives examples of listening to his body-minding brain while exercising his neocortex in such a way as to "manage this great engine of life." This was his way of modeling his path or structure (principle II) for finding "a rational basis, for which the mind hungers" (principle IV), as he stated in chapter 14. His stories also illustrate our need for fellow travelers—some, like Dr. Korr, to serve as role models and others to give us feedback and support as we share ourselves with them. He reminds us that aging is a journey that begins at birth and that the osteopathic principles are a timeless health application of fundamental truths.

As the baby boomers age, more and more books on aging will likely appear to meet the market demand and to quell our fear of aging and ultimately of death.[24] We will all need to be critical evaluators of what medical research presents to us for guidance on healthy aging. Prescriptive advice can quickly become outdated as researchers more fully understand phenomena.[25] Some examples are the changing recommendations on hormone replacement therapy and the ongoing discussions regarding cholesterol and heart disease. Further, anti-aging medicine will continue to develop along with advanced approaches to extending the human life span.[26] It may be difficult for both your healthcare provider and for you to keep up with all the advances, and no less to discern what will be worth the risk and utilization of your resources. Application of these timeless principles, however, will allow you to maintain a healthy bodymind that will give you all the resources you need to meet the future with peace and equanimity. You will be rich no matter what your degree of economic or social "success." How? Let me summarize in very practical terms what Dr. Korr has taught us by his words and by his example.

First, get moving—by whatever means gives you joy. As you start to feel the resistance in your body or in your mind (or in your spirit), LISTEN. What is it saying? Lovingly challenge it. Is it true? Are you absolutely sure it is true?[27] Who or what could assist you in lovingly challenging the barriers, such as, "I don't have time," "I am too old," "I might cause trouble by doing things differently," or "I am comfortable with things as they are."

Next, look at your choices—how you spend your time, what you wear, how you begin or end the day. Would you like to do any of these activities differently? How about the way you greet people or the way you respond to people at work or at home? What would you notice if you did things differently?

While you are doing routine tasks, notice your thoughts. What is passing through your mind? Which thoughts or images keep reoccurring, like a child gently tugging at your sleeve? What is the thought about? What would happen if you paid attention?

Now you are on the path of change. As you continue to listen to your bodymind and spirit, you will be able to listen more effectively to others. What are they saying to you that you couldn't hear before? Does it bring you pain or joy?

Indulge yourself in the freedom of your choices. Notice which choices make you feel joyful. Expand your choices. Move with awareness. Breathe deeply. Notice how each day is a little different. Acknowledge the people around you, whether they are family, friends, or strangers.

As Dr. Korr did, begin to learn about areas that you are unfamiliar with. Learn to do something new. Ask for recommendations from respected experts. The references in this book can be a useful place to begin. Tap into the dreams and visions you had as an adolescent or young adult. How did you see yourself? How could you learn and gather the resources to become that person? To age into your genetic ideal? What path have you been trying to conform to that is not a good "fit" for you? Can you accept your inheritance and develop your God-given gifts?

You don't need much for this journey of health. No expensive equipment or membership card. All you need is around you—your family and friends. (If you are not connected to a support system, you need to make amends with the people who love you.) With the ground at your feet and the wind at your back, you just need to begin.

Dr. Korr very eloquently articulated these ideas in 1999 when he said, "Having lived according to the laws of nature, I can expect to die young—when I am very old."

The references at the end of this epilogue provide sources where you can find more in-depth information about osteopathic principles, the history of osteopathy, and the current status of research in the field. In appendix 3, there is a list of the US state associations of osteopathic medicine and worldwide osteopathic organizations that can assist you in locating an osteopathic physician.

NOTES

1. E. R. Booth, *History of Osteopathy* (Cincinnati: Caxton Press, 1924), p. 435; A. T. Still, *Philosophy of Osteopathy* (Kirksville, MO: 1899), p. 79; G. Webster, *Sage Sayings of Still* (Los Angeles: 1935), p. 25.

2. A. T. Still, *Autobiography of Andrew T. Still* (Kirksville, MO: 1908), pp. 358, 369.

3. *Journal of the American Osteopathic Association* 8 (1908): 3; Andrew Taylor Still papers, 2.2:56; Andrew Taylor Still papers, 2.2:46; A. T. Still, *Research and Practice* (Kirksville, MO: 1910), p. 25.

4. J. Crosby, "The Road to Be Taken: AOA Leadership on Complementary and Alternative Medicine," *D.O.* (June 2001): 11–12.

5. B. Peterson, ed., *The Collected Papers of Irvin M. Korr* (Colorado Springs, CO: American Academy of Osteopathy, 1979); H. H. King, ed., *The Collected Papers of Irvin M. Korr*, vol. 2 (Indianapolis: American Academy of Osteopathy, 1997).

6. K. Kinsella and V. A. Velkoff, *An Aging World: 2001* (Washington, DC: US Census Bureau, Series P95/01-1, 2001).

7. J. J. McGovern, "Osteopathically Caring for the Old," *Still University Review* (Fall 2006): 5–6 (repr. from the *German Journal of Osteopathy*); R. J. McGovern, "Aging and Osteopathy: The Role of Evidence," *Still University Review* (Fall 2006): 10–13 (repr. from the *German Journal of Osteopathy*).

8. J. J. McGovern and R. J. McGovern, *Your Healer Within: A Unified Field Theory of Healthcare* (Tucson: Fenestra, 2003); J. J. McGovern and R. J. McGovern, "The Evolution of the Mind-Body-Spirit Unit," in *Morphodynamics in Osteopathy*, ed. T. Liem (Hamburg: Hippokrates Thieme Enke, 2006), pp. 141–47.

9. J. W. Atchison and W. R. English, "Manipulative Techniques for Geriatric Patients," *Manual Medicine* 7 (1996): 825–42; D. Dodson, "Manipulative Therapy for the Geriatric Patient," *Annals of Osteopathic Medicine* 7 (1979): 114–19; C. Hawk et al., "Chiropractic Care for Patients Aged 55 and Older: Report from a Practice-Based Research Program," *Journal of the American Geriatrics Society* 48 (2000): 534–45; V. C. Hoefner, "Osteopathic Manipulative Treatment in Gerontology," *Annals of Osteopathic Medicine* 10 (1982): 546–49; P. E. Kimberly, "Formulating a Prescription for Osteopathic Manipulative Treatment," *Journal of the American Osteopathic Association* 79 (1980): 506–13.

10. M. M. Patterson, "Research in OMT: What Is the Question and Do We Understand It?" *Journal of the American Osteopathic Association* 107 (2007): 8–11.

11. J. Crosby, "Launching an Aggressive Research Agenda: Why Not?"

D.O. (May 2001): 10–11; J. Crosby, "Research and Public Health: New Day Dawns at AOA," *D.O.* (December 2001): 11–12; M. Dyer and D. Wood, "Collaboration on Research Picks up Steam," *Journal of the American Osteopathic Association* 101 (2001): 13–14; S. H. Glover and P. A. Rivers, "Strategic Choices for a Primary Care Advantage: Re-Engineering Osteopathic Medicine for the 21st Century," *Journal of the American Osteopathic Association* 103 (2003): 156–63; J. Goetz, "Rekindling Research," *D.O.* (April 2002): 22–25; J. Goetz, "Research Progress," *D.O.* (April 2002): 26–27; J. Goetz, "Getting Off the Ground," *D.O.* (April 2002): 28–30; V. J. Guillory and G. Sharp, "Research at US Colleges of Osteopathic Medicine: A Decade of Growth," *Journal of the American Osteopathic Association* 103 (2003): 458–59.

12. D. Noll, "Osteopathic Manipulation in the Elderly and Current Clinical Research," *Still University Review* (Fall 2006): 14–19 (repr. from the *German Journal of Osteopathy*).

13. A. G. Chila, "Pneumonia: Helping Our Bodies Help Themselves," *Consultant* (March 1982): 174–88; S. M. Johnson and M. E. Kurtz, "Conditions and Diagnosis for Which Osteopathic Primary Care Physicians and Specialists Use Osteopathic Manipulative Treatment," *Journal of the American Osteopathic Association* 102 (2002): 527–40; C. A. Kline, "Osteopathic Manipulative Therapy, Antibiotics, and Supportive Therapy in Respiratory Infections in Children: Comparative Study," *Journal of the American Osteopathic Association* 63 (1965): 278–81; J. K. Lynch, "Osteopathic Manipulation Treatment in United States Hospitals: Review of the National Hospital Discharge Survey, 1991–1999 (abstract)," (2000); C. Feldman, "Pneumonia in the Elderly," *Clinics in Chest Medicine* 20 (1999): 563–73; J. T. Marrie, "Bronchitis and Pneumonia," in *Infectious Disease in the Aging: A Clinical Handbook*, ed. T. T. Yoshikawa and D. C. Norman (Totowa, NJ: Humana, 2001), pp. 53–65; D. R. Noll et al., "Adjunctive Osteopathic Manipulative Treatment in the Elderly Hospitalized with Pneumonia: A Pilot Study," *Journal of the American Osteopathic Association* 99 (1999): 143–46, 151–52; D. R. Noll et al., "Benefits of Osteopathic Manipulative Treatment for Hospitalized Elderly Patients with Pneumonia," *Journal of the American Osteopathic Association* 100 (2000): 776–82.

14. T. Breithaupt et al., "Thoracic Lymphatic Pumping and the Efficacy of Influenza Vaccination in Healthy Young and Elderly Populations," *Journal of the American Osteopathic Association* 101 (2001): 21–25; E. P. Dugan et

al., "Effect of Lymphatic Pump Techniques on the Immune Response to Influenza Vaccine," *Journal of the American Osteopathic Association* 101 (2001): 472 (abstract); K. M. Jackson et al., "Effect of Lymphatic and Splenic Pump Techniques on the Antibody Response to Hepatitis B Vaccine: A Pilot Study," *Journal of the American Osteopathic Association* 98 (1998): 155–60; D. R. Noll et al., "Effectiveness of a Sham Protocol and Adverse Effects in a Clinical Trial of Osteopathic Manipulative Treatment in Nursing Home Patients," *Journal of the American Osteopathic Association* 104 (2004): 107–13; D. R. Noll et al., "The Effect of Osteopathic Manipulative Treatment on Immune Response to the Influenza Vaccine in Nursing Home Residents: A Pilot Study," *Alternative Therapies in Health and Medicine* 10, no. 4 (2004): 74–76.

15. M. Kuchera and A. W. Kuchera, *Osteopathic Considerations in Systemic Dysfunction* (Kirksville, MO: Kirksville College of Osteopathic Medicine Press, 1990), pp. 33–52; M. R. Wells et al., "Standard Osteopathic Manipulative Treatment Acutely Improves Gait Performance in Patients with Parkinson's Disease," *Journal of the American Osteopathic Association* 99 (1999): 92–98.

16. T. A. Cavalieri et al., "Osteopathic Manipulative Therapy: Impact on Fall Prevention in the Elderly," *Journal of the American Osteopathic Association* 98 (1998): 391 (abstract).

17. P. E. Kimberly, *Somatic Dysfunction Principles of Manipulative Treatment and Illustrative Procedures for Specific Joint Mobilization* (Kirksville, MO: Kirksville College of Osteopathic Medicine, 1980); G. J. D. Bergman et al., "Manipulative Therapy in Addition to Usual Medical Care for Patients with Shoulder Dysfunction and Pain," *Annals of Internal Medicine* 141 (2004): 432–40; J. A. Knebl et al., "Improving Functional Ability in the Elderly via the Spenser Technique, an Osteopathic Manipulative Treatment: A Randomized, Clinical Trial," *Journal of the American Osteopathic Association* 102 (2002): 347–96; D. A. Patriquin, "The Evolution of Osteopathic Manipulative Technique: The Spencer Technique," *Journal of the American Osteopathic Association* 92 (1992): 1134–46; H. Spencer, "Shoulder Technique," *Journal of the American Osteopathic Association* 15 (1916): 218–20.

18. A. K. Daniel, "JAOA Now Requires Public Registration of Clinical Trials," *Journal of the American Osteopathic Association* 107 (2007): 47.

19. H. A. Guess et al., eds., *The Science of the Placebo: Toward an Interdisciplinary Research Agenda* (London: BMJ Books, 2002).

20. N. Gevitz, *The DOs: Osteopathic Medicine in America*, 2nd ed. (Baltimore: Johns Hopkins University Press, 2004).

21. B. Nathan, *Touch and Emotion in Manual Therapy* (New York: Churchill Livingstone, 1999).

22. D. D. Burns, *Feeling Good: The New Mood Therapy* (New York: Avon, 1999); A. Ellis, *Overcoming Destructive Beliefs, Feelings, and Behaviors: New Directions for Rational Emotive Behavior Therapy* (Amherst, NY: Prometheus Books, 2001); A. Ellis and R. A. Harper, *A New Guide to Rational Living* (California: Wilshire, 1977).

23. T. Bennett-Goleman, *Emotional Alchemy: How the Mind Can Heal the Heart* (New York: Harmony Books, 2001), p. 315.

24. W. M. Bortz II, *Dare to Be 100* (New York: Fireside, 1996); S. E. Levkoff, Y. K. Chee, and S. Noguchi, eds., *Aging in Good Health* (Amherst, NY: Prometheus Books, 2003); A. Wil, *Healthy Aging: A Lifelong Guide to Your Physical and Spiritual Well-Being* (New York: Knopf, 2005).

25. J. Le Fanu, *The Rise and Fall of Modern Medicine* (New York: Carroll and Graf, 1999).

26. W. R. Hazzard, "Preventive Gerontology: Edging Ever Closer to the 'Barrier to Immortality,'" *Journals of Gerontology, Series A, Biological Sciences and Medical Sciences* 60 (2005): 594–95; J. E. Morley and L. van den Berg, eds., *Endocrinology of Aging* (Totowa, NJ: Humana, 1999).

27. B. Katie and S. Mitchell, *Loving What Is: Four Questions That Can Change Your Life* (New York: Harmony, 2002).

Appendix 1

THE PROBLEMATIC PARADOX

The Lower the Morbidity, the Lower the Mortality;

The Lower the Mortality, the Higher the Morbidity

This appendix describes one of the most prevalent and fastest-growing problems of our time. While it is felt most deeply by the aged and their families, it must also be confronted by all those who are aging. And who isn't? No small consideration is the enormous impact of an aging population on our national economy. It began insidiously early this century and has swelled to a magnitude that now dominates the national health scene as well as the political and economic scenes. I refer to the unplanned and largely unanticipated exchange that has taken place between the quick and early mortality of the past for the later and long-term morbidity of the present.

Since the beginning of the twentieth century, an unforeseen exchange developed that is the basis of the above paradox. In 1900, about only 4.1 percent of the American people were over sixty-five years of age. Having increased more than three times as fast as the population as a whole, those over the age of sixty-five now represent more than 12.4 percent of the population. It is projected that the percentage will increase to 20 (one in five!) by about the year 2030. Those over eighty-five belong to the most rapidly growing age group.[1]

What accounts for this remarkable accumulation in older people since the beginning of the twentieth century? The answer usually given or assumed is the large increase in life expectancy since 1900, cited at about an increase of thirty years.[2] We have come to assume, and are seldom corrected, that we each have been given a potential gift of thirty years extra to live because the human life span has been increased by that amount.

The facts are quite different. It is not that the human life span has increased but that the average length of life of the general population has increased. It is not that the human race is now living longer but that more of its members are living longer. The error arises when, for convenience, one abbreviates life expectancy at birth, which is the correct term, to life expectancy. The thirty-year increase applies only to the average newborn; the increase in life expectancy of, let us say, a sixty-five-year-old person today is only a fraction of that.

Early in the twentieth century, the chief killers were acute infectious diseases and epidemics. The most numerous victims were infants, children, and young people, and they succumbed in great numbers. Thanks to such factors as improvements in sewerage and sanitation, in living and working conditions, and in nutrition, child labor laws, purer water and pasteurized milk, acquired immunity, decline of virulence of some infectious agents, and even the availability of launderable undergarments, many of these diseases had already begun to decrease in incidence and in killing power by the last decades of the nineteenth century.

The decline continued and accelerated in the twentieth century as the factors listed above continued to improve. There were also improvements in medical care. (I am still discussing the time before the advent of sulfa drugs and antibiotics.) As a result of these numerous factors, infants, children, and youths who would have died under prior conditions now survived those early, more hazardous years to live into adulthood and old age.

A simple example of comparative statistics illustrates what happened. In 1900, one out of ten live-born infants could be expected to die in their first year of life.[3] By midcentury, about three out of one hundred live-born infants could be expected to die in their first year of life.[4] Obviously, this change alone resulted in an enormous statistical increase in life expectancy at birth, specifically in the average age of death of a cohort of newborns. Hence, the first half of the century is epitomized by the first part of the paradox stated in the title of this appendix—the lower the morbidity, the lower the mortality.

An analogy to a hurdle race may further clarify this point. Earlier this century, the first few hurdles in the life span race were quite high, and many runners did not make it over. More recently, these first few hurdles were substantially lowered, so that many more runners have been able to leap over them to the later hurdles and thus to run more of the race. The race itself, however, is not significantly longer, hence the previous statement that it is not so much that people are living longer but that more people are surviving into the later decades.

Unfortunately, the lower mortality and subsequently the increased numbers of people surviving into the later decades have been accompanied by increased morbidity. A few statistics will convey the enormity of the accompanying health problem. Infirmity is rampant in the older population. A large majority, 88 percent or more, of those over sixty-five years of age are victims of one or more chronic diseases of various degrees of severity.[5] For example, 47 percent suffer from arthritis of one kind or another, 34 percent are hypertensive,[6] and almost 25 percent are mentally ill.[7] Also distressingly common in the senior population are cancer, heart disease, stroke, atherosclerosis and impaired peripheral circulation, diabetes, kidney disease, prostatitis and other problems with pelvic organs in both sexes, osteoporosis, various chronic digestive problems, depression, impairments of hearing and vision, neurological syndromes, stiff and painful joints, and other musculoskeletal impairments that limit mobility while increasing social isolation and dependence on others.

The average senior citizen sees physicians more often, is hospitalized twice as often, stays twice as long,[8] and consumes more prescription drugs than those younger than sixty-five.[9] The older person also requires more long-term and costly care. The illnesses of the 12.4

percent of the population who are now sixty-five use 36 percent of spending for healthcare, a significant cost of the nation's total expenditure for healthcare, which at this writing is about to exceed a trillion dollars per year. The total amount spent is almost four billion dollars and is quadruple the personal expenditures for those in the under sixty-five population.[10] The sixty-five-and-older group, who are expected to represent 20 percent of the population around the year 2030, will consume one-half of the nation's expenditure for healthcare, which is expected to exceed two trillion dollars per year by that time. (The coauthor would like to amend that current estimates project healthcare spending in 2015 will exceed four trillion dollars per year.)[11] No wonder that the issue of healthcare for senior citizens has been the subject of intense congressional debate!

No less important are those personal aspects for which there are no quantitative measures, such as the pain, suffering, and dependency of the victims as well as the enormous burdens on families and caregivers. Is there any wonder that some cynical commentators have concluded that a quick and early death is much more merciful to the victim, to the family, and to the national economy than a lingering one?

However, must infirmity increase with age, that is, the older, the sicker? Are the so-called diseases of aging, such as the chronic degenerative diseases, intrinsic and unavoidable aspects of the aging process? Is aging itself pathological? Or, like the infectious diseases that have specific and eradicable causes, are they also subject to cure by finding and eliminating the cause of each disease? Can the chronic diseases also be prevented by some sort of immunization? Or, like the communicable diseases, will they too decline spontaneously as living conditions improve? How do we explain the many thousands who did not and do not succumb to the diseases of aging and who live long, healthy, active lives? Is it entirely a matter of lucky combinations of genes, or is there something about their living conditions that we should examine for possible guidance?

Instead of devoting almost all of our health-related resources to the too-late treatment of established diseases and to the quest for individual causes and cures, we should invest in diminishing and eliminating factors that contribute to vulnerability to diseases in general and especially to the enhancement of health as the most comprehensive form of disease prevention. The sooner and the earlier in life that we begin, the better.

NOTES

1. Administration on Aging, "A Profile of Older Americans: 2005," US Department of Health and Human Services 2005, http://www.aoa.gov/PROF/Statistics/profile/2005/2005profile.pdf (accessed March 19, 2007).

2. National Center for Health Statistics, "Life Expectancy," US Department of Health and Human Services, http://www.cdc.gov/nchs/data/hus/hus06.pdf#027 (accessed March 19, 2007).

3. Morbidity and Mortality Weekly Report, "Achievements in Public Health, 1900–1999: Healthier Mothers and Babies," Centers for Disease Control and Prevention, 1999, http://www.cdc.gov/mmwR/preview/mmwrhtml/mm4838a2.htm (accessed March 19, 2007).

4. Infoplease, "Infant Mortality Rates, 1950–2003," http://www.infoplease.com/ipa/A0779935.html (accessed March 19, 2007).

5. J. L. Wolff, "Prevalence, Expenditures, and Complications of Multiple Chronic Conditions in the Elderly," *Archives of Internal Medicine* 162 (2002): 2269–76.

6. "Chronic Conditions among the Elderly in the United States," ASCP Professional Affairs Department, http://www.ascp.com/resources/clinical/upload/ (accessed March 19, 2007).

7. "Mental Health of the Elderly," American Psychiatric Association, http://healthyminds.org/mentalhealthofelderly.cfm (accessed March 19, 2007).

8. C. J. DeFrances, M. N. Podgornik, and Division of Health Care Statistics, "2004 National Hospital Discharge Survey," Advance Data from Vital and Health Statistics 2006, http://www.cdc.gov/nchs/data/ad/ad371.pdf (accessed March 19, 2007).

9. "Medications and Older People," US Food and Drug Administration, http://www.fda.gov/fdac/features/1997/697_old.html (accessed March 20, 2007).

10. S. P. Keehan et al., "Age Estimates in the National Health Accounts," *Health Care Financing Review*, http://www.cms.hhs.gov/NationalHealth ExpendData/downloads/keehan-age-estimates.pdf (accessed March 20, 2007).

11. K. Davis et al., "Slowing the Growth of US Health Care Expenditures: What Are the Options?" Commonwealth Fund, January 2007, http://www.cmwf.org/usr_doc/Davis_slowinggrowthUShltcareexpenditureswhat areoptions_989.pdf (accessed March 20, 2007).

Appendix 2
SUPPLEMENT TO CHAPTER 13
Other Systems Controlled by the Body-Minding Brain

RESPIRATION

The respiratory center, located in the hindbrain or brain stem, is the oldest part of the body-minding brain, which tails off into the spinal cord. The more recently evolved pons and midbrain (see figure 2 of the photo insert) operate in such a manner that oxygen is supplied to the body as rapidly as it is consumed, and carbon dioxide is eliminated from the body as rapidly as it is produced. Under most conditions, adjustment of pulmonary ventilation according to the carbon dioxide concentration in the blood ensures, at the same time, adequate delivery of oxygen. The primary respiratory center in the medulla oblongata is especially sensitive to carbon dioxide, and its discharge of impulses to the respiratory muscles fluctuates with changes in its concentration. In other words, the higher the concentration, the faster the ventilation. Since carbon dioxide becomes carbonic acid when dissolved in an aqueous medium, the respiratory system also has an important role in acid-base regulation.

As is true of most biological control mechanisms, there is, fortunately, a backup system. The backup mechanism in respiratory control is sensitive to oxygen concentration in the blood. It becomes particularly important in conditions in which oxygen supply is reduced, such as at high altitudes, when the breath is held, or when the carbon dioxide mechanism does not meet oxygen requirements. Under these conditions, the hypoxic (low oxygen) mechanisms take over, calling for deeper and more rapid breathing, even though this results in "blowing off" carbon dioxide. These backup mechanisms involve sensory receptors that are sensitive to hypoxemia (low oxygen concentration in the blood). The most important ones are strategically located in the aorta, the body's main artery, and in the carotid arteries, which carry blood to the brain and other structures in the head.

In addition, the respiratory centers are responsive to sensory reports from other parts of the body. Receptors in the lungs report their degree of distention with each inhalation and play a role in the regulation of depth and rate of respiration. Reports from receptors as well as metabolic products in the musculoskeletal system seem to be important in the adjustment of breathing during physical activity. The respiratory centers, like the cardiovascular centers and others (see below), are also under the influence of higher centers that summon resources in anticipatory warm-up for such exertions as flight from predators, pursuit of prey, or climbing a long flight of stairs.

CIRCULATION OF THE BLOOD

While the machinery of the circulatory system is different from that of the respiratory system, the principles of control are the same. The cardiovascular centers, relying on feedback from various reporting stations and on chemical cues, control the amount of blood pumped per minute by the heart, called the cardiac output, by regulating the force and volume of each beat and the number of beats per minute. The centers also control the resistance to blood flow by regulating the internal diameters of the chief resistance vessels, namely, the arterioles. These arterioles are the minutest of the arterial branches, which, in turn, branch profusely to form the capillaries.

It is across the thin, highly permeable capillary walls that oxygen, nutrients, and other essential substances move from blood to cells and across which products of metabolism and special cellular products move from cells to blood for distribution or disposal. Blood flow through the capillaries must, at all times, be adequate to meet the logistical requirements of every cell. Moreover, the flow must be within a narrow range of pressures sufficient to cause adequate filtration across the capillary walls but not so high as to cause edema (fluid accumulation in the tissues).

If the total resistance offered by the arterioles is too high, as in hypertension, then the heart must be driven by the brain centers to create and maintain a high enough pressure in the arteries to force adequate flow to all the tissues. Producing this high arterial pressure is very costly to the heart. If it is maintained too long, it may damage not only the heart but also the arteries, the brain, the kidneys, and other organs. Therefore, the regulation of arterial blood pressure is another major responsibility of the centers in the brain.

By controlling arteriolar resistance in each tissue, the centers and local chemical factors control distribution of the cardiac output according to the changing relative and individual needs of all the tissues and organs. Blood, like electricity, follows the path of least resistance. At a given arterial pressure, blood flow through each tissue will vary inversely as the resistance. Thus, when we are physically active, blood is shunted to the active muscles by dilatation of their arterioles, and cardiac output is increased to maintain an adequate flow to all the tissues. After a heavy meal, vascular resistance in the gastrointestinal tract is lowered, increasing blood flow for digestion and absorption. Similarly, in hot weather, blood flow through the skin must be substantially increased to promote the transfer of heat to the environment. Such preferential diversion of blood must, furthermore, be accomplished while maintaining adequate flow to all other parts of the body, particularly to the part most vulnerable to oxygen privation—the brain.

These are but a few of the ways in which the brain directs and coordinates the components of the cardiovascular system in meeting the logistical needs of every part of the body under widely and rapidly varying circumstances, with maximum efficiency and minimum cost, and while assigning top priority to itself.

OTHER HOMEOSTATIC CONTROLS

I trust that these few examples give the reader a fairly representative notion of the ways in which body-minding parts of the brain do indeed care for the body. We need say less perhaps about others, such as the control of fluid volumes, electrolyte content, food intake, digestion, acid-base balance, metabolic level, body weight, sleep, and such defensive responses as coughing, sneezing, and vomiting.

Unlike the controls discussed above, which go on automatically and reflexively, controls of fluid volume and of food consumption require active participation by the animal or the person in the form of drinking and eating and in the cessation of each. Thus, we are alerted to the need for replenishment of evaporated or excreted water by sensory reports of dryness in the mouth. Their volleys of impulses to the brain are experienced by us as thirst. We are still not sure, scientifically speaking, where the signal "enough" originates; it certainly is given long before the water has been absorbed.

While experience shows that the thirst mechanism is quite reliable in the control of water intake, the control of fluid volumes and of the concentrations of the various electrolytes is a great deal more complex. Control includes that of distribution of fluids among the various compartments, such as blood, lymph, cerebrospinal fluid, intracellular and intercellular fluids, and so on, and control of their respective electrolyte composition. Adjustments are made in accordance with the feedback provided by numerous reporting stations in the body. These controls require, in addition to the reflex mechanisms, the participation of the endocrine glands (pituitary and adrenal cortex) and, of course, the kidneys and their neural and endocrine regulation. Incidentally, secretion by the pituitary is controlled by the hypothalamus through direct neural connections. The pituitary, in turn, hormonally controls other endocrine glands, including the adrenal cortex.

Appendix 3

RESOURCES FOR FINDING OSTEOPATHIC HEALTH PROFESSIONALS

T he following is a list of resources for locating an osteopathic health professional in your area; it is organized in two sections by resources in the United States and the rest of the world. For resources within the United States, the listing progresses alphabetically by state. An additional resource for interested readers would be the American Osteopathic Association, which can be contacted at: AOA Main Headquarters, 142 East Ontario Street, Chicago, IL 60611; toll-free phone: (800) 621-1773; general phone: (312) 202-8000; fax: (312) 202-8200; Web site: http://www.osteopathic.org.

OSTEOPATHIC HEALTH PROFESSIONALS IN THE UNITED STATES

An asterisk (*) after a listing indicates that particular Web site contains a physician directory.

ALABAMA

Alabama Osteopathic Medical Association, Tuscaloosa
(205) 487-7556
E-mail: dr_hatfield@hotmail.com

ALASKA

Alaska Osteopathic Medical Association
(972) 416-8727
E-mail: hmacriss@osteopathic.org

ARIZONA

Arizona Osteopathic Medical Association,* Phoenix
(602) 266-6699
E-mail: mweaver@az-osteo.org

ARKANSAS

Arkansas Osteopathic Medical Association, Little Rock
(501) 374-8900
E-mail: osteomed@ipa.net

CALIFORNIA

Osteopathic Physicians and Surgeons of California,* Sacramento
(916) 561-0724
E-mail: opsc@opsc.org

COLORADO

Colorado Society of Osteopathic Medicine, Denver
(303) 322-1752
E-mail: marie@coloradodo.org

CONNECTICUT

Connecticut Osteopathic Medical Society, Avon
(800) 648-9777
E-mail: ptortland@jockdoctors.com

DELAWARE

Delaware State Osteopathic Medical Society, Wilmington
(302) 764-1198
E-mail: info@deosteopathic.org

DISTRICT OF COLUMBIA

Osteopathic Association of the District of Columbia, Arlington
(703) 522-8404

FLORIDA

Florida Osteopathic Medical Association, Tallahassee
(850) 878-7364
E-mail: admin@foma.org

GEORGIA

Georgia Osteopathic Medical Association, Tucker
(770) 493-9278
E-mail: exdir@goma.org

HAWAII

Hawaii Association of Osteopathic Physicians and Surgeons,
    Honolulu
(800) 891-0333
E-mail: hmacriss@osteopathic.org

ILLINOIS

Illinois Osteopathic Medical Society, Chicago
(312) 202-8174
E-mail: ioms@ioms.org

INDIANA

Indiana Osteopathic Association, Indianapolis
(317) 926-3009
E-mail: mclaphan@aol.com

IOWA

Iowa Osteopathic Medical Association, Des Moines
(515) 283-0002
E-mail: leah@ioma.org

KANSAS

Kansas Association of Osteopathic Medicine, Topeka
(785) 234-5563
E-mail: kansasdo@aol.com

KENTUCKY

Kentucky Osteopathic Medical Association, Frankfort
(502) 223-5322
E-mail: info@koma.org

LOUISIANA

Louisiana Osteopathic Medical Association
(318) 385-7943
E-mail: loma@osteopathic.org

MAINE

Maine Osteopathic Association, Manchester
(207) 623-1101
E-mail: kmiller@mainedo.org

MARYLAND

Maryland Association of Osteopathic Physicians, Baltimore
(410) 683-8100
E-mail: maops@maops.com

MASSACHUSETTS

Massachusetts Osteopathic Society, Inc., Winchester
(800) 621-1773, ext. 8164
E-mail: massachusetts@osteopathic.org

MICHIGAN

Michigan Osteopathic Association, Okemos
(800) 657-1556
E-mail: moa@mi-osteopathic.org

MINNESOTA

Minnesota Osteopathic Medical Society, Lakeland
(612) 623-3268
E-mail: colleenjensen@pressenter.com

MISSISSIPPI

Mississippi Osteopathic Medical Association, Jackson
(601) 366-3105
E-mail: info@moma-net.org

MISSOURI

Missouri Association of Osteopathic Physicians and Surgeons, Inc.,
    Jefferson City
(573) 634-3415
E-mail: contact@maops.org

MONTANA

Montana Osteopathic Association*
(701) 852-8798
E-mail: cbell@ndak.net

NEBRASKA

Nebraska Association of Osteopathic Physicians and Surgeons,
    Omaha
(800) 617-5310
E-mail: mbatchelder@osteopathic.org

NEVADA

Nevada Osteopathic Medical Association, Henderson
(702) 434-7112
E-mail: nvoma@earthlink.net

NEW HAMPSHIRE

New Hampshire Osteopathic Association, Concord
(603) 224-1909
E-mail: joy.potter@nhms.org

NEW JERSEY

New Jersey Association of Osteopathic Physicians and Surgeons,
    Monmouth Junction
(732) 940-9000
E-mail: rbowen@njosteo.com

NEW MEXICO

New Mexico Osteopathic Medical Association, Albuquerque
(505) 332-2146
E-mail: admin@nmoma.org

NEW YORK

New York State Osteopathic Medical Society, Inc.
(800) 841-4131
E-mail: nysoms@nysoms.org

NORTH CAROLINA

North Carolina Osteopathic Medical Association, Wilmington
(888) 626-6248
Fax: (910) 763-4666
E-mail: ncoma@ncoma.org

NORTH DAKOTA

North Dakota State Osteopathic Association
(701) 852-8798
E-mail: ndoma@ndoma.org

OHIO

Ohio Osteopathic Association,* Columbus
(614) 299-2107
E-mail: jwills@ooanet.org

OKLAHOMA

Oklahoma Osteopathic Association,* Oklahoma City
(405) 528-4848
E-mail: ooa@okosteo.org

OREGON

Osteopathic Physicians and Surgeons of Oregon, Portland
(503) 222-2779 or (800) 533-6776
E-mail: jeffh@opso.org

PENNSYLVANIA

Pennsylvania Osteopathic Medical Association, Harrisburg
(717) 939-9318
E-mail: poma@poma.org

RHODE ISLAND

Rhode Island Society of Osteopathic Physicians and Surgeons
(781) 721-9900 or (800) 454-9663
E-mail: nocdos@comcast.net

SOUTH CAROLINA

South Carolina Osteopathic Medical Society
(800) 621-1773, ext. 8162
E-mail: southcarolina@osteopathic.org

SOUTH DAKOTA

South Dakota Osteopathic Association, Sioux Falls
(605) 338-3427

TENNESSEE

Tennessee Osteopathic Medical Association, Nashville
(615) 345-9550
E-mail: jallen@xmi.us.com

TEXAS

Texas Osteopathic Medical Association,* Austin
(512) 708-8662 or (800) 444-8662
E-mail: toma@txosteo.org

UTAH

Utah Osteopathic Association, Payson
(801) 465-9545
E-mail: uoma@qwest.net

VERMONT

Vermont State Association of Osteopathic Physicians and Surgeons,
    Inc., Montpelier
(802) 229-9418 or (800) 454-9663
E-mail: nocdos@comcast.net

VIRGINIA

Virginia Osteopathic Medical Association
(804) 334-4655
E-mail: voma@voma-net.org

WASHINGTON

Washington Osteopathic Medical Association, Inc.,* Seattle
(206) 937-5358
E-mail: kitter@woma.org

WEST VIRGINIA

West Virginia Society of Osteopathic Medicine, Inc., Charleston
(304) 345-9836
E-mail: wvdo@wvsominc.org

WISCONSIN

Wisconsin Association of Osteopathic Physicians and Surgeons,
    Racine
(262) 619-9901
E-mail: waops1@yahoo.com

WYOMING

Wyoming Association of Osteopathic Physicians and Surgeons
(602) 266-5698
E-mail: hmacriss@osteopathic.org

MILITARY PERSONNEL

Association of Military Osteopathic Physicians & Surgeons
(410) 519-8217
E-mail: jyonts@amops.org

OSTEOPATHIC HEALTH PROFESSIONALS OUTSIDE THE UNITED STATES

AUSTRALIA

Australian Osteopathic Association
http://www.osteopathic.com.au/

CANADA

Canadian Osteopathic Association (COA)
http://www.osteopathic.ca/

Canadian Osteopathic Association, Calgary, Alberta
(403) 282-7165
E-mail: tfindlay@telus.net

GERMANY

Deutsch-Amerikanischen Akademie für Osteopathie DAAO e.V.
http://www.daao.info/

INTERNATIONAL

Osteopathic International Alliance
http://www.oialliance.org/

World Osteopathic Health Organization (WOHO)
http://www.woho.org/

ACKNOWLEDGMENTS

DR. IRVIN M. KORR

There are many people to thank for contributing, directly and indirectly, to this book. Most prominent in my mind are the following, identified more or less in chronological order.

Morris Thompson, president emeritus of the Kirksville College of Osteopathic Medicine, who, on the recommendation of the late, distinguished neuroscientist Professor Ralph M. Gerard, MD, PhD, invited me in 1945 to embark on a professional adventure that absorbs and excites me to this day. I would also like to thank Professor Gerard, who persuaded me to accept the invitation.

The late Margot Lindsay Korr, who, at great cost to herself, joined and staunchly supported me in this adventure until her death in January 1975.

The late John A. Chace, DO, for teaching me that my options were open with respect to my health and for introducing me to the "physician within" with wonderful and enduring effect.

Physician-colleagues at the Kirksville, Michigan State University, and University of North Texas colleges of osteopathic medicine who, through

their care, taught me much about their clinical philosophy, art, and science, and who helped me meet my responsibility to the physician within.

I want to thank all those who, having heard my lectures on healthy
aging, encouraged me to write this book.

My wife, Janet, who made this book possible through her loving
support and helpful criticism, and by the very ambiance that she creates
in our home. The photographic illustrations are also her contribution.

My son, David, for *his* support and professional criticism. I wish I
could learn and put into practice all that he could teach me about
writing.

Frank Manci, who, with the skill and dedication of a great teacher,
introduced this reluctant pupil, at the age of eighty-one, to the world
of computers and word processing.

Those who read earlier drafts and made valid criticisms and
helpful suggestions: Frances Townsend, Mary Folsom, Steven Jonas,
MD, and, especially Patty Meneley, for skilled and sensitive editing
while improving my computer competence.

DR. RENE J. McGOVERN

There are many people to thank. First, I would like to thank Steven L.
Mitchell, editor in chief at Prometheus Books. I am honored and proud
to be, along with Dr. Korr, a member of the Prometheus family. Great
thanks also to A. T. Still University (ATSU) and, in particular my husband, James J. McGovern, president of ATSU. Without his support, this
project would not have been possible. Special thanks to Jason Haxton,
director of the Still Osteopathic Museum, for unearthing the manuscript,
recognizing its importance, and linking Jan Korr and myself to undertake publication. Special thanks also to Jan Korr for her faith in me as
well as her support and insight into her husband's work.

There are numerous others, of course, without whom this work
would not have been possible: Deb Goggin for her extensive editorial
assistance; Dena Higbee for her hours spent working with Jason

Haxton on scanning the manuscript to convert it into electronic format; Pamela Bosch, PhD, PT, associate professor of physical therapy, and Alison Snyder, PhD, ATC, assistant professor of interdisciplinary health sciences and clinical education coordinator in the athletic training program, for their professional insight into exercise in chapters 11 and 12; associate dean Stephen Laird, DO, and chairman of the Neurobehavioral Sciences Department, G. Barry Robbins, DO, for giving me release time to work on the manuscript; and last but definitely not least, Debbie Kelly, who initially spent hours correcting the scanned document and later made sure that my time was truly protected by watching over my patients and my academic responsibilities with great care so that I was assured nothing was neglected.

I would be remiss if I did not end by thanking my parents, Louis and Lucille Pugliese, who are models of healthy aging and inspire me daily.

GLOSSARY

acidosis or alkalosis. Respectively, high pH or low pH, referring to a measure of the acidity of a substance. See also **pH**.

adipose tissue. Technical term used in anatomy to refer to body fat.

adrenal cortex. The portion of the adrenal gland that mediates the stress response through the production of mineralocorticoids and glucocorticoids, including aldosterone and cortisol.

aerobic exercise. Physical activity that can be continued at a more or less steady pace for an extended period of time. Aerobic exercise includes such activities as walking, jogging, cross-country skiing, swimming, cycling, dancing, rowing, and rope skipping. In physiological terms, the energy for these kinds of activities is derived from oxidation of glucose and other substances within the muscle fibers themselves. The increased volumes of oxygen are delivered by increased ventilation of the lungs through deeper and more rapid breathing and by increased pumping action of the heart with a subsequent widening of blood vessels in the active muscles.

ameliorative change. Introduction of positive change or removal of negative precursors.

asphyxiation. A lack of oxygen to the body from being unable to breathe normally.

261

autonomic nervous system (ANS) or visceral nervous system. A part of the peripheral nervous system that controls homeostasis. It does so by controlling cardiovascular, digestive, and respiratory functions and also salivation, perspiration, diameter of the pupils, micturition (the discharge of urine), and erection. Most of the activities of the ANS are involuntary; however, some functions, such as breathing, can be in part consciously controlled, making the "autonomic nervous system" not completely autonomous.

baby boomer. Term used to refer to the demographic group of people born during the post–World War II period and before the Vietnam War. This large cohort has had a disproportionate influence on demographic trends.

basal metabolic rate. The speed of metabolism, which influences how much food an organism will require.

Benson, Herbert (1935–). American cardiologist and founder of the Mind/Body Medical Institute near Boston, Massachusetts. A graduate of Harvard Medical School, Dr. Benson defined the *relaxation response* and led teaching and research into its efficacy in counteracting the harmful effects of stress.

Bierce, Ambrose Gwinnett (June 24, 1842–1914?). American satirical writer and journalist, best known for his *Devil's Dictionary.*

Billings, Josh (April 20, 1818–October 14, 1885). Humorist and lecturer whose birth name was Henry Wheeler Shaw. He was a contemporary of Mark Twain.

Bismarck, Otto von. Chancellor of Germany in 1889 credited with setting the retirement age at sixty-five. The chancellor arbitrarily used the life expectancy of the time, age forty-three, and added half that number, setting the eligibility for pensions at age sixty-five. That age continues to this day to be the age for retirees to begin receiving benefits, despite significant increases in life expectancy.

body armor, or bodymind armor. The natural guarding response of our musculature to emotional trauma; considered to be fundamentally the same as that to the threat of physical trauma.

bodymind. Term used to express the oneness of body and mind, as opposed to mind-body dualism.

body's own pharmacy. Metaphor for the biochemicals that are produced by the body to promote healing.

Borysenko, Joan. Cofounder and former director of the Mind/Body Clinical Programs at the Beth Israel Deaconess Medical Center, Harvard Medical School. She has a doctorate in medical sciences from Harvard Medical School, is a licensed clinical psychologist, and is currently the president of Mind/Body Health Sciences, Inc. Her area of specialty is women's health and spirituality, integrative medicine, and the mind/body connection. She is the author of *Minding the Body, Mending the Mind.*

calorie. The amount of heat required to raise the temperature of one milliliter of water by one degree Celsius.

Cannon, Walter B. Harvard physiologist who, in 1915, coined the term *fight or flight* in describing an animal's response to threats. He also developed the concept of homeostasis and popularized it in his book *The Wisdom of the Body*, published in 1932.

cantilever. A beam supported at one end with the other end projecting into space. Cantilever construction allows for overhanging structures without using external bracing.

cantilever bridge. A bridge built using cantilevers, which project horizontally into space, supported on only one end.

carnivores. Animals whose diet consists mainly of meat, whether it comes from living animals or dead ones (scavenging). (Latin *carne* meaning flesh and *vorare* meaning to devour.)

causes of health. The various protective, immunological, detoxifying, healing, recuperative, restorative, regenerative, compensatory, and regulatory homeostatic mechanisms. Also included is the understanding of the comprehensive protective role of the brain as director and coordinator of these mechanisms as well as of our behavior.

caveat. From the Latin word *cavere* meaning "warning" (or more literally, "let him beware"); included in Latin phrases such as *caveat* *lector* (let the reader beware) or *caveat emptor* (let the buyer beware).

cerebral cortex. A structure within the vertebrate brain that plays a central role in many complex brain functions including memory, attention, perceptual awareness, "thinking," language, and consciousness.

cilia. Microscopic whiplike structures in the lining of the respiratory tubing.

Cognitive Behavioral Therapy (CBT). A widely used psychotherapy that developed out of behavior modification and cognitive therapy, based on the premise that feelings and behavior result from how individuals think about themselves and their lives. A significant body of research has supported the efficacy of CBT for many disorders, including mood disorders, anxiety disorders, and adjustment to major changes in life. CBT has been administered in both individual and group formats and with self-help manuals and, increasingly, self-help software packages.

cohort. A group of people who share a particular statistical or demographic characteristic (e.g., birth, graduation, job loss, exposure to a drug or a vaccine, etc.).

Complementary and Alternative Medicine (CAM). Alternative medicine describes practices used in place of conventional medical treatments. Complementary medicine describes practices used in conjunction and cooperation with conventional medicine to assist the existing process. The term *complementary and alternative medicine* (CAM) is an umbrella term for both branches. CAM includes practices that incorporate spiritual, metaphysical, or religious underpinnings; nonevidence-based practices; non-European medical traditions; or newly developed approaches to healing.

connective tissue. The supporting or framework tissue of the animal body formed of fibrous and ground substance with numerous cells of various kinds. The varieties of connective tissue are areolar or loose; adipose; dense, regular or irregular, white fibrous; elastic; mucous; lymphoid tissue; cartilage; and bone. The blood and lymph may also be regarded as connective tissues.

consensus trance. Term used to connote a nonreflective, habitual way of viewing reality and unquestioned beliefs. Attributed to experimental psychologist Charles T. Tart, PhD.

constitutional differences. Human variation believed to be based on genetic inheritance as contrasted to environmental influences.

Cooper, Kenneth H. (1931–). Physician and author of the 1968 book *Aerobics*, which emphasized a point system for improving the cardiovascular system, which is the basis of the ten thousand steps per day method of maintaining adequate fitness by walking. Dr. Cooper is the founder of the Cooper Aerobics Center in Dallas, Texas.

coup de grâce. French for "blow of mercy." A death blow intended to end the suffering of a wounded creature. It is often used figuratively to describe the last of a series of events that brings about the end of some entity.

Cousins, Norman (June 24, 1915–November 30, 1990). A prominent political journalist, author, and world peace advocate, who also served as adjunct professor of medical humanities for the School of Medicine at the University of California. Cousins did research on the biochemistry of human emotions, which he long believed were the key to human beings' success in fighting illness. Late in life Cousins was diagnosed with a form of arthritis then called Marie-Strumpell's disease. He described his struggle with this illness in the book *Anatomy of an Illness*.

Darwin, Charles Robert (February 12, 1809–April 19, 1882). English naturalist who convinced the scientific community that species develop over time in a process of evolution. His theories of natural and sexual selection are central to the modern evolutionary synthesis as the unifying theory of the life sciences, especially biology but also in other disciplines, such as anthropology, psychology, and philosophy.

decrepitude. Decrease in functional ability usually attributed to aging.

degenerative disorders. Diseases of the musculoskeletal system and connective tissue.

Descartes, René (1596–1650). French philosopher-scientist to whom the concept that the body and the mind are two separate and independent domains is usually attributed.

diaphragm. In mammals, a shelf of muscle extending across the bottom of the rib cage. The diaphragm separates the thoracic cavity (with lung and heart) from the abdominopelvic cavity (with liver, stomach, intestines, etc.). In its relaxed state, the diaphragm is shaped like a dome. It is controlled by the phrenic nerve. In order to avoid confusion with other types of diaphragm, it is sometimes referred to as the thoracic diaphragm. Any reference to the diaphragm in this text is understood to refer to this structure.

digoxin. A cardiac medication extracted from the foxglove plant, *Digitalis lanata*. Digoxin is widely used in the treatment of various heart conditions, namely, atrial fibrillation, atrial flutter, and congestive heart failure.

dualistic thinking. Approach to organizing reality that categorizes information into one of only two possible alternatives—black and white, either-or thinking.

electrolyte balance. The regulation of the osmotic pressure of body fluids to maintain the homeostasis of the body's water content and keep the body's fluids from becoming too dilute or too concentrated. In physiology, a significant electrolyte disturbance usually constitutes a medical emergency. Severe or prolonged electrolyte disturbance can lead to cardiac problems, neuronal malfunction, organ failure, and ultimately death.

endocoids. Term coined by Harbans Lal, PhD, to describe the large and diverse pharmacy of the body's own medicines. Examples of endocoids are those substances that are manufactured in various parts of the brain and are called neuropeptides, such as the endorphins.

endocrine glands. Glands that have no ducts, their secretions being absorbed directly into the blood.

endogenously. Originating or produced within the organism or one of its parts.

endorphin. Neuropeptide produced by the brain that is chemically related to morphine.

enzyme. A protein that acts as a catalyst to induce chemical changes in other substances, itself remaining apparently unchanged by the process. Enzymes, with the exception of those discovered long ago (e.g., pepsin, emulsin), are generally named by adding -*ase* to the name of the substrate on which the enzyme acts (e.g., glucosidase), the substance activated (e.g., hydrogenase), and/or the type of reaction (e.g., oxidoreductase, transferase, hydrolase, lyase, isomerase, ligase, or synthetase—these being the seven main groups in the Enzyme Nomenclature Recommendations of the International Union of Biochemistry).

eugeriatrics. A term coined by Irvin M. Korr for aging that is healthy or gives one a feeling of fulfillment; the art and science of healthy aging.

eustress. A term referring to stress that has positive benefits for health and well-being.

facilitated (hyperexcitable) segment. That part of the nervous system where patterns of sensory nerve impulses or feedback sent by affected joints, muscles, ligaments, and tendons are exaggerated or garbled so that an "irritable focus" is established. Since there is no way that the central nervous system can organize an adaptive response to such unintelligible signals, it calls for what amounts to a holding pattern. The result is the immobilization of that part of the body due to the sustained muscular contraction.

fight-or-flight response. Acute stress response of animals and the first stage of the general adaptation syndrome (GAS). This includes a discharge of the sympathetic nervous system, preparing the animal for fighting or fleeing. The fight-or-flight response was first described by Walter B. Cannon in 1927.

food additives. Substances added to food to preserve flavor or improve its taste and appearance. Some additives have been used for centuries; for example, preserving food by pickling (with vinegar), salting, as with bacon, or using sulfur dioxide as in some wines. With the advent of processed foods in the second half of the twentieth century, many more additives have been introduced, of both natural and artificial origin. Also included are various preservatives; herbicides; pesticides; insecticides; antibiotics; hormones; fertilizers; artificial flavoring, coloring, and sweeteners; salt; and other minerals. Some of them are known to be carcinogenic or hazardous to our health in other ways, especially when repeatedly consumed over long periods of time. The effects some of them have on our bodies and our overall health have yet to be determined.

Friedan, Betty (February 4, 1921–February 4, 2006). American feminist, activist, and writer. She is best known for her book *The Feminine Mystique*, which articulated the discontent of women in the 1950s and initiated the "Second Wave" of feminism.

gastroenterology. The branch of medicine that specializes in the care of the digestive system including the gastrointestinal tract (i.e., organs from mouth to anus). The term comes from the Greek words *gastros* (stomach), *enteron* (intestine), and *logos* (reason). Specialists in the field are called gastroenterologists.

gastrointestinal system (GI tract). The organ system within multicellular animals that takes in food, digests it to extract energy and nutrients, and expels the remaining waste. Other terms include digestive tract, alimentary canal, or gut.

General Adaptation Syndrome (GAS). A systemic adaptive response to prolonged stress, involving alarm, resistance, exhaustion. Attributed to Hans Selye, a Canadian endocrinologist.

Goethe, Johann Wolfgang von (August 28, 1749–March 22, 1832). German poet, dramatist, novelist, theorist, humanist, scientist, and painter. He is considered a giant of the literary world. His most enduring work and a masterpiece of world literature is the two-part dramatic poem *Faust*. Goethe's other well-known works include *Wilhelm Meister's Apprenticeship*, the novel *The Sorrows of Young Werther*, and the semiautobiographical novella *Elective Affinities*, which was one of the first texts to speculate on the nature of interpersonal chemistry.

health. Wholeness; total intactness of the person—mind, body, and spirit.

herbivores. Any organism that eats only plants.

high-level health/wellness. Progress toward higher potentials of functioning; a continual challenge to live at a fuller potential; the integration of the total individual in body, mind, and spirit in the functioning process.

Hippocrates (c. 460 BCE–c. 370 BCE). Ancient Greek physician, often referred to as the "Father of Medicine" and considered an important figure in the history of medicine. The Hippocratic school of medicine revolutionized medicine in ancient Greece by establishing it as a discipline distinct from other fields that it had traditionally been associated with (notably theurgy and philosophy).

HIV (human immunodeficiency virus). A retrovirus that causes acquired immunodeficiency syndrome (AIDS).

homeokinesis. Term coined by Irvin M. Korr to replace the term *homeostasis* to represent the dynamic quality of the thousands of body systems that maintain equilibrium within the body.

homeostasis. The state of equilibrium (balance between opposing pressures) in the body with respect to various functions and to the chemical compositions of the fluids and tissues. The processes through which such bodily equilibrium is maintained.

hominids. Any member of the biological family Hominidae (the "great apes"). This includes the humans, chimpanzees, gorillas, and orangutans.

hormones. Chemical substances formed in the body and transported by the blood to specific organ or body parts; depending on the specificity of their effects, hormones can alter the functional activity or the structure of just one organ or tissue or various numbers of them. Estrogen, insulin, secretin, cholecystokinin, and pancreozymin, formed in the gastrointestinal tract, are examples of hormones.

human ceiling. Physiologic limits at which humans can perform successfully.

hyperglycemia. Abnormally high concentration of glucose in the blood, seen especially in patients with diabetes.

hyper- or hypotension. Respectively, high blood pressure or low blood pressure.

hyper- or hypothermia. Respectively, high body temperature or low body temperature.

hypoglycemia. Abnormally low levels of glucose in the blood. Normal glucose range is 60–100 mg/dL (3.3–5.6 mmol/L). The resulting symptoms are either autonomic, including sweating, trembling, feelings of warmth, anxiety, and nausea, or neuroglycopenic symptoms, which include feelings of dizziness, confusion, tiredness, difficulty speaking, headache, and inability to concentrate.

hypoxia. Decrease below normal levels of oxygen in inspired gases, arterial blood, or tissue, short of anoxia.

idiopathic. Adjective used to describe a disease or constellation of symptoms that arise spontaneously or from an obscure or unknown cause.

idiosyncratic. A structural or behavioral characteristic peculiar to an individual or group.

immobilization. Inability to move.

immune system. Mechanisms within an organism that protect against infection by identifying and killing pathogens, distinguishing them from the organism's normal cells and tissues. Detection is complicated as pathogens adapt and evolve new ways to successfully infect the host organism.

infirmity. A weakness; an abnormal, more or less disabling condition of mind or body.

inflammatory processes. Also referred to as immune mediated inflammatory disease (IMID); a group of conditions or diseases that are the result of a dysregulation of the normal immune response leading to inflammation. The inflammation can cause organ damage and is associated with increased morbidity and/or mortality. Inflammation is the primary driver of many diseases, including ankylosing spondylitis, psoriasis, psoriatic arthritis, Behçet's disease, arthritis, inflammatory bowel disease (IBD), autoimmune diseases, and allergy as well as many of the cardiovascular, neuromuscular, and infectious diseases. Some current research suggests that uncontrolled inflammatory processes are responsible for aging.

integrative medicine. Healthcare that combines mainstream medical therapies and complementary and alternative medical (CAM) therapies for which there is some evidence of safety and effectiveness.

interactive unity. Osteopathic principle that indicates that each aspect of a human being interacts with all other aspects; interaction of mind, body, and spirit.

interferons (IFNs). Proteins belonging to a class of gycoproteins known as cytokines, which are produced by the immune system in response to foreign agents such as viruses, bacteria, parasites, and tumor cells, and which assist the immune response by inhibiting viral replication within other cells of the body.

interleukins. A group of cytokines, or signaling molecules, that are key to immune function. They were first identified in white blood cells (leukocytes, hence the -*leukin*) but subsequently were found to be produced by a wide variety of bodily cells. Deficiency in interleukins has been identified in autoimmune diseases or immune deficiency.

internist. Physicians who specialize in nonsurgical diseases in adults, not including diseases limited to the skin or to the nervous system.

interstitial fluid. The internal environment of the cells consisting of thin fluid layers that bathe the cells. This is essentially a filtrate of blood plasma with the filtration taking place across the capillary walls.

Koop, C. Everett (October 14, 1916–). American physician who served as the surgeon general of the United States from 1982 to 1989.

Kuhn, Maggie (August 3, 1905–April 22, 1995). Lifelong American activist most famous for founding the Gray Panthers movement in 1971 after being forced into retirement by the Presbyterian Church. The Gray Panthers advocated nursing home reform and fought ageism, claiming that "old people constitute America's biggest untapped and undervalued human energy source." She dedicated her life to fighting for human rights, social and economic justice, global peace, integration, and an understanding of mental health issues. Four years after writing her autobiography, *No Stone Unturned*, she died of cardiopulmonary arrest in Philadelphia at the age of 89.

Law of Fixity—Fluxity. Concept used by Irvin M. Korr to help students understand homeostasis as a manifestation of the dynamic balance of constancy, or fixity, of levels as being due to a dynamic balance between opposite fluxes, or changes. The mental image he used for these processes was that of a rapidly flowing mountain stream whose level at each point is constant because outflow is balanced by inflow from the source.

ligament. A term used in anatomy to denote three different types of structures: 1. fibrous tissue that connects bones (or two different parts of a single bone), sometimes called articular ligaments, fibrous ligaments, or rue ligaments; 2. a fold of peritoneum or other membrane; or 3. the remnant of a tubular structure from the fetal period. Reference in this book is to the first and most common usage of the term.

mammalian species. A class of vertebrate animals characterized by the production of milk in females for the nourishment of young; the presence of hair or fur; specialized teeth; three small bones in the ear; the presence of a neocortex region in the brain; endothermic, or "warm-blooded," bodies; and, in most cases, the existence of a placenta.

medical physiology. Application of the science concerning the normal vital processes of animal and vegetable organisms to medical care, especially as to how things normally function in the living organism rather than to their anatomical structure, their biochemical composition, or how they are affected by drugs or disease.

Medicare. A publicly funded health insurance program in the United States, generally for the elderly and disabled.

Menninger, Karl Augustus (July 22, 1893–July 18, 1990). American psychiatrist and cofounder with his father of the Menninger Foundation and the Menninger Clinic, a psychiatric and psychoanalytic center in Topeka, Kansas. After World War II, Menninger was instrumental in founding the Winter Veterans Administration Hospital in Topeka, which became the largest psychiatric training center in the world.

mind-muscle interplay. Belief that changing mental and emotional tensions, both the pleasant and the unpleasant, are accompanied by corresponding patterns of muscular tension; chronic tensions and unresolved emotional conflicts are reflected in sustained muscular contractions that may have deleterious consequences, such as pain, weakness, and fatigue.

morbidity. A diseased state. The ratio of sick to well in a community. The frequency of the appearance of complications following a surgical procedure or other treatment. The term *morbidity rate* can refer either to the incidence rate or to the prevalence rate of a disease. Compare this with the mortality rate of a condition, which is the number of people dying during a given time interval, divided by the total number of people in the population. Morbidity is often what is measured by intensive care unit (ICU) scoring systems.

musculoskeletal system. Relating to muscles and to the skeleton; the part of the human body that comprises the muscles, bones, joints, ligaments, tendons, and other connective tissues.

myth of health versus disease. Belief that health and illness are fixed, either-or entities rather than existing on a continuum.

National Center for Complementary and Alternative Medicine (NCCAM). A division of the US National Institutes of Health (NIH) created to evaluate and disseminate scientific evidence evaluating the effectiveness of complementary and alternative healing practices. NCCAM defines complementary and alternative medicine as "a group of diverse medical and healthcare systems, practices, and products that are not presently considered to be part of conventional medicine."

National Institute on Aging (NIA). A division of the National Institutes of Health established in 1974 to improve the health and well-being of older Americans through research on aging.

National Institutes of Health (NIH). An agency of the US Department of Health and Human Services responsible for biomedical research with the goal of acquiring new knowledge to help prevent, detect, diagnose, and treat disease and disability.

natural defensive mechanisms. Bodily mechanisms that protect us against poisonous and harmful chemicals we ingest with our food and drink or absorb through our skin and lungs. This mechanism works in several ways. For instance, the immune system disarms foreign proteins while the liver, kidneys, and intestinal tract convert those proteins into harmless substances and eliminate them from the body.

neocortex. A part of the brain exclusively in mammals. The neocortex is part of the cerebral cortex (along with the archicortex and paleocortex, which are cortical parts of the limbic system) involved in higher functions such as sensory perception, generation of motor commands, spatial reasoning, conscious thought, and in humans, language.

nephrology. Derived from the Greek word *nephros*, which means kidney; the branch of internal medicine dealing with the study of the function and diseases of the kidney.

nervous system. The organ system that includes the brain, the spinal cord, and an enormous network of nerves throughout the body. The nervous system is responsible for coordinating the activity of the muscles, monitoring the organs, constructing and inhibiting input from the senses, and initiating actions.

neuropeptides. Any of a variety of peptides found in neural tissue, for example, endorphins and enkephalins. These are products of the body's own pharmacy that are manufactured in various parts of the brain. Some of the best-known neuropeptides are the endorphins, chemical cousins of morphine.

neurotransmitter. Any specific chemical agent (including acetylcholine, five amines, four amino acids, two purines, and more than twenty-eight peptides) released by a presynaptic cell upon excitation that crosses the synapse to stimulate or inhibit the post-synaptic cell. More than one may be released at any given synapse. The neurotransmitters released by presynaptic cells may modulate transmitter release from presynaptic cells.

New York Academy of Sciences. A society of over twenty thousand scientists of all disciplines from 150 countries whose mission is "to advance the understanding of science, technology, and medicine, and to stimulate new ways to think about how their research is applied in society and the world." The membership of the New York Academy of Sciences has included Nobel Prize winners and notable people such as Thomas Jefferson, James Monroe, Charles Darwin, John James Audubon, and Albert Einstein.

normal. A statistical reference to data that lack significant deviation from the average or middle of the bell-shaped curve. Root word for *abnormal*, having a negative connotation and sometimes indicating illness or pathology.

omnivore. Animals that are able to eat and digest both plant and animal matter.

orthopedics or orthopedic surgery (also spelled orthopaedics). The branch of medicine that treats disorders of the musculoskeletal system, including arthritis, trauma, and congenital deformities.

paradigm. Term used since the late 1960s in reference to the set of assumptions, concepts, values, and practices that predominate in any intellectual discipline. A set way of viewing reality.

parasympathetic nervous system. A division of the autonomic nervous system that conserves energy by slowing the heart rate, increasing intestinal and gland activity, and relaxing sphincter muscles in the gastrointestinal tract. The sympathetic and parasympathetic divisions of the nervous system complement each other, with the sympathetic division preparing the organism for "fight or flight" and the parasympathetic conserving the necessary energy for the organism to continue to function once it is no longer in danger.

Pasteur, Louis (December 27, 1822–September 28, 1895). A French chemist known for his breakthroughs in microbiology that confirmed the germ theory of disease and developed the field of bacteriology. He is best known for developing the process of pasteurization, which was utilized to stop milk and wine from going sour.

peripheral nerves. Those nerves that deliver impulses and neurotransmitters to the tissues and organs of the body. They also supply the trophic (nurturing) proteins that are manufactured in the nerve cells.

pH. The measure of acidity or alkalinity of a solution. A pH less than seven is considered acidic, while a pH of greater than seven is basic (alkaline).

physical medicine and rehabilitation (PM&R), or physiatry. A branch of medicine that specializes in the functional restoration of people affected by physical disability. Physicians who complete the specialized training, which includes one year of internship and a three-year residency, are called physiatrists.

physician within. Metaphor for the mechanisms that produce the biochemicals responsible for healing.

placebo. Latin word meaning "I will please." An inert compound identical in appearance to material being tested in experimental research, which may or may not be known to the physician and/or patient, administered to distinguish between drug action and suggestive effect of the material under study.

postnatal development. Development of the human infant that takes place after birth.

primates. In biological classification, the group that contains the species related to the lemurs, monkeys, and apes, which also includes humans.

prostaglandins. Member of a group of lipid compounds derived enzymatically from fatty acids that have important functions in the animal body. Every prostaglandin contains twenty carbon atoms, including a five-carbon ring. Prostaglandins act as mediators and have a variety of strong physiological effects; although technically hormones, they are rarely classified as such.

psyche. The Greek word for "soul," currently applied to the modern ideas of soul, self, and mind. The root for the term *psychology*, study of the soul.

psychoneuroimmunology (PNI). Field of research developed in the 1970s that studies the interactions between social psychology, behavior, the brain, and the immune system. More recently the importance of the endocrine system was noted and the field's name changed to psychoneuroendoimmunology (PNEI). Scientific research in PNEI investigates the effects of the "mind-body" interactions in both health and disease in all fields of medicine: pediatrics, psychiatry, internal medicine, gastroenterology, obstetrics, gynecology, orthopedics, and cardiology. The field also investigates malfunctions of the neuroimmune system in disorders (autoimmune diseases, hypersensitivities, immune deficiency) and the physical, chemical, and physiological characteristics of the components of the neuroimmune system.

psychosomatic medicine. Field of medicine developed to address the growing recognition in the healing professions that what goes on in the mind (psyche) has powerful influences on what goes on in the body (soma), and that there are psychological effects of physical activities and illnesses.

quadruped. Term used to refer to land animals that use four legs for locomotion.

reductionism. Scientific or research viewpoint that believes the way to understand humans and their frailties is to take them apart and reduce them to their component parts.

respiratory muscles. Muscles that assist in effective breathing, including the intercostals (between the ribs), the accessory muscles, the diaphragm, and the muscles of the abdomen. The respiratory muscles, like other skeletal muscles, are subject to conscious and deliberate control.

sacrum. Large, triangular bone, inserted like a wedge between the two hip bones, at the base of the spine and at the upper and back part of the pelvic cavity.

Selye, Hans Hugo Bruno (born Selye János, January 26, 1907–October 16, 1982). Canadian endocrinologist who contributed important theoretical work on the nonspecific response of the organism to stress. Selye is considered the first to demonstrate the existence of the stress syndrome, or general adaptation syndrome (GAS).

Shambhala meditation. A secular approach to meditation that draws its name from the legend of Shambhala, an ancient Asian kingdom where all members of the society were said to be enlightened. Shambhala teachings focus on the inherent dignity and goodness of people and encourage students to cultivate bravery and gentleness in order to expose their hearts to the world. Shambhala meditation was developed by the late Vidyadhara Chögyam Trungpa Rinpoche and his students.

sine qua non. Latin for "without which it could not be," or an indispensable and essential action, condition, or ingredient. The phrase is in general use in many languages, including English, German, French, and Italian, with applications in economics, philosophy, and medicine.

Social Security. A field of social welfare service, originally established by Franklin D. Roosevelt in 1935 in the United States, that utilizes federal resources for individual protection against social conditions, including poverty, old age, disability, and unemployment.

sociocultural environment. Influence on the individual by the social culture in which they live. This includes language, history, social customs, and the influence of the natural environment within which they developed.

somatic. Relating to the soma or trunk, the wall of the body cavity, or the body in general; the skeletal (voluntary) muscles and their innervation, as distinct from the viscera or visceral (involuntary) muscle and its (autonomic) innervation.

somatoemotional release. The reported experience of osteopathic physicians and other manual therapists that, while manipulatively unraveling a knot in a patient's body, a release of emotions, which manifest in tears, anger, or painful memories, occurs. This phenomenon can be understood as a long-blocked healing process of bodymind being released. It has been described by Jack Painter, PhD, as a breach of the bodymind armor.

sports medicine. An interdisciplinary healthcare subspecialty, including but not restricted to specialty physicians and surgeons, athletic trainers, physical therapists, coaches, and, of course, the athlete, that deals with the treatment and preventive care of athletes, both amateur and professional.

statistical man. Use of the statistical average in laboratory and other biomedical measures to identify "normal" and prescribe without taking individual human diversity into account. Professor Roger J. Williams made the challenge in a talk to the National Academy of Sciences in 1955 and in his book *Biochemical Individuality* that the statistical man has no counterpart in a population of real individuals.

stress. Reactions of the body to forces of a deleterious nature, infections, and various abnormal states that tend to disturb its normal physiologic equilibrium (homeostasis).

subjacent. Underlying.

sympathetic nerves or sympathetic nervous system (SNS). The part of the autonomic nervous system (ANS) responsible for neuronal and hormonal activation, commonly known as the fight-or-flight response. It does so by mediating complex homeostatic mechanisms that regulate up or down in living organisms. Activation of the sympathetic nervous system impacts functions such as pupil diameter, gut motility, and urinary output. This response is also known as the sympathoadrenal response of the body, since it also involves the secretion of acetylcholine from the adrenal medulla, which activates the secretion of adrenaline (epinephrine) and to a lesser extent noradrenaline (norepinephrine).

tendons. Fibrous tissue designed to withstand tension that connects muscle to bone or muscle to muscle. Ligaments are similar to tendons but they join one bone to another.

Thomas, Lewis (November 25, 1913–December 3, 1993). Physician, poet, etymologist, essayist, administrator, educator, policy advisor, and researcher whose autobiography, *The Youngest Science: Notes of a Medicine Watcher*, is a record of a century of medicine and the changes that occurred in it. He won a National Book Award in 1974 for a collection of essays titled *The Lives of a Cell.*

Type A personality. A set of characteristics that includes being impatient, excessively time conscious, insecure about one's status, highly competitive, hostile and aggressive, and incapable of relaxation. The type B personality, in contrast, is patient, relaxed, and easygoing. There is also a type AB mixed profile for people who have a combination of both types of personality.

unity of the body. Used to indicate that every part of the body is in communication with every other part through the circulating blood and the nervous system.

unity of the person. Used to indicate union of the body, mind, and spirit; conveys the idea of a totally integrated humanity and individuality.

variometer. An instrument in an aircraft used to inform the pilot of the rate of descent or climb.

vertebrae. Individual bones that make up the vertebral or spinal column. There are usually thirty-three vertebrae in humans, including the five that are fused to form the sacrum (the others are separated by intervertebral discs) and the four coccygeal bones that form the tailbone.

verticality. Upright stance.

viscera. Reference to the internal organs, that is, the heart, lungs, kidneys, and so on.

visceral functions. The purposeful activities of the internal organs, such as peristalsis, cardiac output, or kidney function. What internal organs do.

vis medicatrix naturae. Ancient Latin phrase that indicates the early awareness of the importance of nature's healing power within each of us. Ultimately healing occurs through the enormously complex biological mechanisms subsumed under *vis medicatrix naturae.*

vulnerability. Susceptibility to physical or emotional injury or attack.

whole-person context. Approach to research that includes the many varying features and modifying circumstances unique to the human species and human life, and those unique to the individual person, including the unique manner in which individuals respond and adapt to those circumstances. Utilization of the whole-person context completes the reductionistic paradigm.

Williams, Roger J. (August 14, 1893–February 20, 1988). Professor and biochemist, known for writing the widely read book *Biochemical Individuality*, who named folic acid and discovered pantothenic acid.

World Health Organization (WHO). Agency of the United Nations, with headquarters in Geneva, Switzerland, established in 1948 that acts as a coordinating authority on international public health. It was preceded by the Health Organization, an agency of the League of Nations.

YMCA (Young Men's Christian Association, or "the Y"). A worldwide social movement founded in London, England, in 1844, by Sir George Williams in response to the unhealthy social conditions in London at the end of the Industrial Revolution. The YMCA uses a holistic approach to individual and social development of young people with a mission of building a healthy spirit, mind, and body.

yoga. One of the six schools of Hindu philosophy, focusing on meditation as a path to self-knowledge and personal freedom. Among the Hindu texts attributed to establishing the basis for yoga are the *Upanishads*, the *Bhagavad Gita*, the *Yoga Sutras of Patanjali*, and the *Hatha Yoga Pradipika*. In India, yoga is seen as a means to physiological and spiritual mastery. Outside India, yoga has become primarily associated with the practice of asanas or postures, although it has influenced spiritual practices throughout the world. A dedicated practitioner of yoga is referred to as a yogi, yogin (masculine), or yogini (feminine). Yoga as a combination of mental, spiritual, and physical exercises has been practiced for more than five thousand years.

yoga as exercise. While yoga evolved as a spiritual practice, in the West it has grown popular as a form of purely physical exercise. Some Western yoga practice has little to do with Hinduism or spirituality, but is simply a way of keeping fit and healthy. This differs from the traditional Eastern view of yoga, although it is not always possible to separate completely "exercise yoga" from "spiritual yoga." Yoga was introduced to American society in the late nineteenth century by Swami Vivekananda, the founder of the Vedanta Society.

YWCA (Young Women's Christian Association). A women's membership movement founded in England in 1855 that strives to create opportunities for women's growth, leadership, and power in order to eliminate racism and empower women. The YWCA is independent of the YMCA.

SOURCES FOR THE GLOSSARY

Stedman's Online Medical Dictionary (http://stedmans.com)
Wikipedia Online Encyclopedia (http://en.wikipedia.com)

BIBLIOGRAPHY

Achterberg, J. *Imagery in Healing: Shamanism and Modern Medicine.* Boston: New Science Library, 1985.

Ader, R., N. Cohen, and D. L. Felten, eds. *Brain, Behavior and Immunity.* Vol. 3. New York: Academic Press, 1989.

———, eds. *Psychoneuroimmunology.* 3rd ed. 2 vols. San Diego: Academic Press, 2001.

Administration on Aging. "A Profile of Older Americans: 2005." US Department of Health and Human Services 2005. http://www.aoa.gov/PROF/ Statistics/profile/2005/2005profile.pdf (accessed March 19, 2007).

American College of Sports Medicine. *ACSM's Guidelines for Exercise Testing and Prescription.* 7th ed. Philadelphia: Lippincott Williams and Wilkins, 2005.

———. "Exercise and Physical Activity for Older Adults." *Medicine and Science in Sports and Exercise* 30 (1998): 992–1008.

American Dietetic Association. "American Dietetic Association Home Page." http://www.eatright.org/cps/rde/xchg/ada/hs.xsl/index.html (accessed March 28, 2007).

American Society for Clinical Pathology (ASCP) Professional Affairs Department. "Chronic Conditions among the Elderly in the United States." http://www.ascp.com/resources/clinical/upload/ (accessed March 19, 2007).

Anderson, B. *Stretching*. Bodinas, CA: Shelter, 1980.

———. *Stretching*. Rev. ed. Bolinas, CA: Shelter, 2000.

Andrews, H. F. "Helping and Health: The Relationship between Volunteer Activity and Health-Related Outcomes." *Advances* 7 (1990): 25–34.

Andrew Taylor Still papers. 2.2:46 and 2.2:56.

Atchison, J. W., and W. R. English. "Manipulative Techniques for Geriatric Patients." *Manual Medicine* 7 (1996): 825–42.

Beasley, J. D. *The Betrayal of Health*. New York: Times Books, 1991.

Ben-Ari, M. *Just a Theory: Exploring the Nature of Science*. Amherst, NY: Prometheus Books, 2005.

Bennett-Goleman, T. *Emotional Alchemy: How the Mind Can Heal the Heart*. New York: Harmony Books, 2001.

Benson, H., and M. Z. Klipper. *The Relaxation Response*. New York: Avon, 1976.

Berger, P. B. "New Directions in Research: Report from the 10th International Conference on AIDS." *Canadian Medical Association Journal* 152 (1995): 1991–95.

Bergman, G. J. D., J. C. Winters, K. H. Groenier, J. J. Pool, B. Meyboom-de Jong, K. Postema, and G. J. van der Heijden. "Manipulative Therapy in Addition to Usual Medical Care for Patients with Shoulder Dysfunction and Pain." *Annals of Internal Medicine* 141 (2004): 432–40.

Berland, T. *Fitness for Life: Exercises for People over 50*. Washington, DC: American Association of Retired Persons, 1986.

Bierce, A. *The Devil's Dictionary*. Mount Vernon, NY: Peter Pauper, 1958.

Billings, J. *Josh Billings, Hiz Sayings*. Kila, MT: Kessinger, 2006.

Blair, S. N., J. B. Kampert, H. W. Kohl III, C. E. Burlau, C. A. Macera, R. S. Paffenbarger Jr., and L. W. Gibbons. "Influences of Cardiorespiratory Fitness and Other Precursors on Cardiovascular Disease and All-Cause Mortality in Men and Women." *Journal of the American Medical Association* 276 (1996): 205–10.

Booth, E. R. *History of Osteopathy*. Cincinnati: Caxton Press, 1924.

Borrell-Carrio, F., A. L. Suchman, and R. M. Epstein. "The Biopsychosocial Model 25 Years Later: Principles, Practice, and Scientific Inquiry." *Annals of Family Medicine* 2 (2004): 576–82.

Bortz, W. M., II. *Dare to Be 100*. New York: Fireside, 1996.

———. "Disuse and Aging." *Journal of the American Medical Association* 248 (1982): 1203–1208.

————. "Geriatrics: Through the Looking Glass." *Medical Times* (June 1989): 85–92.

Borysenko, J. *Minding the Body, Mending the Mind.* Reading, MA: Addison-Wesley, 1987.

Breithaupt, T., K. Harris, J. Ellis, E. Purcell, J. Weir, M. Clothier, and D. Boesler. "Thoracic Lymphatic Pumping and the Efficacy of Influenza Vaccination in Healthy Young and Elderly Populations." *Journal of the American Osteopathic Association* 101 (2001): 21–25.

Brody, H. *Stories of Sickness.* New York: Oxford University Press, 2003.

Brody, H., and D. Brody. *The Placebo Response.* New York: HarperCollins, 1997.

————. *The Placebo Response.* Rev. ed. New York: Cliff Street, 2000.

Brody, J. *Jane Brody's Nutrition Book.* New York: Norton, 1981.

Browning, R. "Rabbi Ben Ezra." In *Robert Browning*, edited by A. Roberts. Oxford: Oxford University Press, 1997.

Burns, D. D. *Feeling Good: The New Mood Therapy.* New York: Avon, 1999.

Calvin, W. H. *A Brief History of the Mind: From Apes to Intellect and Beyond.* New York: Oxford University Press, 2004.

Cannon, W. B. *Wisdom of the Body.* Gloucester, MA: Peter Smith, 1963.

Caporale, L. H. *Darwin in the Genome: Molecular Strategies in Biological Evolution.* New York: McGraw-Hill, 2003.

Cavalieri, T. A., D. L. Miceli, M. Goldis, E. V. Masterson, L. Forman, and S. C. Pomerantz. "Osteopathic Manipulative Therapy: Impact on Fall Prevention in the Elderly." *Journal of the American Osteopathic Association* 98 (1998): 391 (abstract).

Charnetski, C., and F. X. Brennan. *Feeling Good Is Good for You.* New York: St. Martin's, 2001.

Chila, A. G. "Pneumonia: Helping Our Bodies Help Themselves." *Consultant* (March 1982): 174–88.

Chopra, D. *Perfect Health.* New York: Three Rivers Press, 2000.

————. *Quantum Healing: Exploring the Frontiers of Mind/Body Medicine.* New York: Bantam, 1989.

Christensen, A. *Easy Does It Yoga.* New York: Fireside, 1999.

Christensen, A., and D. Rankin. *Easy Does It Yoga for Older People.* San Francisco: Harper and Row, 1979.

Churchill, J. D., R. Galvez, S. Colcombe, R. A. Swain, A. F. Kramer, and W. T. Greenough. "Exercise, Experience and the Aging Brain." *Neurobiology of Aging* 23 (2002): 941–55.

Cohen, S. "Social Support and Physical Illnesses." *Advances* 7 (1990): 35–47.

Colbert, D. *Deadly Emotions: Understand the Mind-Body-Spirit Connection That Can Heal or Destroy You*. Nashville: Nelson Books, 2003.

Conner, S. L., and W. E. Conner. *The New American Diet*. New York: Simon and Schuster, 1986.

Cooper, K. *Running Without Fear*. New York: M. Evans, 1985.

Cousins, N. *Anatomy of an Illness as Perceived by the Patient*. New York: Norton, 1979.

———. *The Healing Heart*. New York: Norton, 1983.

Crosby, J. "Launching an Aggressive Research Agenda: Why Not?" *D.O.* (May 2001): 10–11.

———. "Research and Public Health: New Day Dawns at AOA." *D.O.* (December 2001): 11–12.

———. "The Road to Be Taken: AOA Leadership on Complementary and Alternative Medicine." *D.O.* (June 2001): 11–12.

Crowley, C., and H. S. Lodge. *Younger Next Year for Women*. New York: Workman, 2005.

Daniel, A. K. "JAOA Now Requires Public Registration of Clinical Trials." *Journal of the American Osteopathic Association* 107 (2007): 47.

Darwin, C., J. Moore, and A. Desmond. *The Descent of Man*. New York: Penguin Classics, 2004.

Davis, K., C. Schoen, S. Guterman, T. Shih, S. C. Schoenbaum, and I. Weinbaum. "Slowing the Growth of US Health Care Expenditures: What Are the Options?" Commonwealth Fund, January 2007. http://www.cmwf .org/usr_doc/Davis_slowinggrowthUShltcareexpenditureswhatare options_989.pdf (accessed March 20, 2007).

DeFrances, C. J., M. N. Podgornik, and Division of Health Care Statistics. "2004 National Hospital Discharge Survey." Advance Data from Vital and Health Statistics 2006. http://www.cdc.gov/nchs/data/ad/ad371.pdf (accessed March 19, 2007).

Demasio, A. R. *Descartes' Error: Emotion, Reason, and the Human Brain*. New York: Putnam, 1994.

Depp, C. A., and D. V. Jeste. "Definitions and Predictors of Successful Aging: A Comprehensive Review of Larger Quantitative Studies." *American Journal Geriatric Psychiatry* 14 (2006): 6–20.

Deutsch, D. *The Fabric of Reality*. New York: Penguin, 1998.

Dodson, D. "Manipulative Therapy for the Geriatric Patient." *Annals of Osteopathic Medicine* 7 (1979): 114–19.

Dubos, R. *Mirage of Health: Utopias, Progress and Biological Change.* New York: Harper, 1959.

Duff, G. W. "Evidence for Genetic Variation as a Factor in Maintaining Health." *American Journal of Clinical Nutrition* 83 (2006): 431S–435S.

Dugan, E. P., W. W. Lemley, C. A. Roberts, M. Wager, and K. M. Jackson. "Effect of Lymphatic Pump Techniques on the Immune Response to Influenza Vaccine." *Journal of the American Osteopathic Association* 101 (2001): 472 (abstract).

Dunn, H. L. *High-Level Wellness.* Arlington, VA: R. W. Beatty, 1961.

———. *Your World and Mine.* 2nd ed. New York: Exposition, 1956.

Duyff, R. L. *American Dietetic Association Complete Food and Nutrition Guide.* 3rd ed. New York: Wiley, 2006.

Dychtwald, K., ed. *Wellness and Health Promotion for the Elderly.* Rockville, MD: Aspen, 1986.

Dyer, M., and D. Wood. "Collaboration on Research Picks up Steam." *Journal of the American Osteopathic Association* 101 (2001): 13–14.

Eccles, J. C. *Evolution of the Brain: Creation of the Self.* New York: Routledge, 1989.

Eisenberg, D. M., R. C. Kessler, C. Foster, F. E. Norlock, D. R. Calkins, and T. L. Delbanco. "Unconventional Medicine in the United States: Prevalence, Costs, and Patterns of Use." *New England Journal of Medicine* 328 (1993): 246–52.

Ellis, A. *Overcoming Destructive Beliefs, Feelings, and Behaviors: New Directions for Rational Emotive Behavior Therapy.* Amherst, NY: Prometheus Books, 2001.

Ellis, A., and R. A. Harper. *A New Guide to Rational Living.* Chatsworth, CA: Wilshire, 1977.

Engel, G. "The Clinical Application of the Biopsychosocial Model." *American Journal of Psychiatry* 137 (1980): 534–44.

———. "The Need for a New Medical Model: A Challenge for Biomedicine." *Science* 196 (1977): 129–36.

Erikson, E. H., J. M. Erikson, and H. Q. Kivnick. *Vital Involvement in Old Age.* New York: Norton, 1986.

Fabre, C., K. Chamari, P. Mucci, J. Massé-Biron, and C. Préfaut. "Improvement of Cognitive Function by Mental and/or Individualized Aerobic

Training in Healthy Elderly Subjects." *International Journal of Sports Medicine* 23 (2002): 415–21.

FallCreek, S., and M. Mettler. *A Healthy Old Age: A Sourcebook for Health Promotion with Older Adults*. Rev. ed. New York: Haworth, 1984.

Farfan, H. F. "The Biomechanical Advantage of Lordosis and Hip Extension for Upright Activity: Man as Compared with Other Anthropoids." *Spine* 3 (1978): 336–42.

Farquhar, J. W. *The American Way of Life Need Not Be Hazardous to Your Health*. New York: Norton, 1978.

Feldman, C. "Pneumonia in the Elderly." *Clinics in Chest Medicine* 20 (1999): 563–73.

Fleg, J. L., C. H. Morrell, A. G. Bos, L. J. Brant, L. A. Talbot, J. G. Wright, and E. G. Lakatta. "Accelerated Longitudinal Decline of Aerobic Capacity in Healthy Older Adults." *Circulation* 112 (2005): 674–82.

Frankel, R. M., T. E. Quill, and S. H. McDaniel, eds. *The Biopsychosocial Approach: Past, Present, and Future*. Rochester, NY: University of Rochester Press, 2003.

Freier, S., ed. *The Neuroendocrine-Immune Network*. Boca Raton, FL: CRC Press, 1989.

Friedan, B. *The Fountain of Age*. New York: Simon and Schuster, 1993.

Fries, J. F. *Aging Well*. Reading, MA: Addison-Wesley, 1989.

———. "Aging, Illness, and Health Policy: Implications of the Compression of Morbidity." *Perspectives in Biology and Medicine* 31 (1988): 407–28.

Furst, A. "Can Nutrition Affect Chemical Toxicity?" *International Journal of Toxicology* 21 (2002): 419–24.

Gevitz, N. *The DOs: Osteopathic Medicine in America*. 2nd ed. Baltimore: Johns Hopkins University Press, 2004.

Glatt, S. J., P. Chayavichitsilp, C. Depp, N. J. Schork, and D. V. Jeste. "Successful Aging: From Phenotype to Genotype." *Biological Psychiatry* 62, no. 4 (2007): 282–93.

Glover, S. H., and P. A. Rivers. "Strategic Choices for a Primary Care Advantage: Re-Engineering Osteopathic Medicine for the 21st Century." *Journal of the American Osteopathic Association* 103 (2003): 156–63.

Goethe, J. W., and J. P. Eckermann. *Conversations of Goethe with Johann Peter Eckermann*. Translated by J. Oxenford and edited by J. K. Moorhead. New York: Da Capo, 1998.

Goetz, J. "Getting off the Ground." *D.O.* (April 2002): 28–30.

———. "Rekindling Research." *D.O.* (April 2002): 22–25.

———. "Research Progress." *D.O.* (April 2002): 26–27.

Goldberg, E. *The Wisdom Paradox: How Your Mind Can Grow Stronger as Your Brain Grows Older.* New York: Gotham, 2005.

Goldstritch, J. D. *Best Chance Diet.* Atlanta: Humanics, 1982.

Green, E., and A. Green. *Beyond Biofeedback.* New York: Delta, 1975.

Greenspan, S. I., and S. G. Shanker. *The First Idea: How Symbols, Language, and Intelligence Evolved from Our Primate Ancestors to Modern Humans.* Cambridge, MA: Da Capo, 2004.

Guess, H. A., L. Engel, A. Kleinman, and J. Kusek, eds. *The Science of the Placebo: Toward an Interdisciplinary Research Agenda.* London: BMJ Books, 2002.

Guillory, V. J., and G. Sharp. "Research at US Colleges of Osteopathic Medicine: A Decade of Growth." *Journal of the American Osteopathic Association* 103 (2003): 458–59.

Gulati, M., D. K. Pandey, M. F. Arnsdorf, D. S. Lauderdale, R. A. Thisted, R. H. Wicklund, A. J. Al-Hani, and H. R. Black. "Exercise Capacity and the Risk of Death in Women: The St. James Women Take Heart Project." *Circulation* 108 (2003): 1554–59.

Hall, S. S. "A Molecular Code Links Emotions, Mind, and Health." *Smithsonian* 20 (1989): 62–71.

Harris, G. *Body and Soul.* New York: Kensington, 1999.

Hawk, C., C. R. Long, K. T. Boulanger, E. Morschhauser, and A. W. Fuhr. "Chiropractic Care for Patients Aged 55 and Older: Report from a Practice-Based Research Program." *Journal of the American Geriatrics Society* 48 (2000): 534–45.

Hayflick, L. *How and Why We Age.* New York: Ballantine, 1994.

Hazzard, W. R. "Preventive Gerontology: Edging Ever Closer to the 'Barrier to Immortality.'" *Journals of Gerontology. Series A, Biological Sciences and Medical Sciences* 60 (2005): 594–95.

———. "Preventive Gerontology. Strategies for Healthy Aging." *Postgraduate Medicine* 74 (1983): 279–87.

Hazzard, W. R., J. P. Blass, W. H. Ettinger, J. B. Halter, and J. G. Ouslander. *Principles of Geriatric Medicine and Gerontology.* 4th ed. New York: McGraw-Hill, 2000.

"Healthy People 2010 Spotlight." National Center for Health Statistics. http://www.cdc.gov/nchs/hphome.htm (accessed March 23, 2007).

Hirshberg, C., and M. I. Barasch. *Remarkable Recovery: What Extraordinary Healings Tell Us about Getting Well and Staying Well.* New York: Riverhead, 1995.

Hodes, R. J., V. Cahan, and M. Pruzan. "The National Institute on Aging at Its Twentieth Anniversary: Achievements and Promise of Research on Aging." *Journal of the American Geriatrics Society* 44 (1996): 204–206.

Hoefner, V. C. "Osteopathic Manipulative Treatment in Gerontology." *Annals of Osteopathic Medicine* 10 (1982): 546–49.

Holmes, T. H., and R. H. Rahe. "The Social Readjustment Rating Scale." *Journal of Psychosomatic Research* 11 (1967): 213–18.

House, J. S., K. R. Landis, and D. Umberson. "Social Relationships and Health." *Science* 241 (1988): 540–45.

Hrøbjartssøn, A., and P. C. Gøtzsche. "Is the Placebo Powerless? An Analysis of Clinical Trials Comparing Placebo with No Treatment." *New England Journal of Medicine* 344 (2001): 1594–1602.

Infoplease. "Infant Mortality Rates, 1950–2003." http://www.infoplease.com/ipa/A0779935.html (accessed March 19, 2007).

Jackson, K. M., T. F. Steele, E. P. Dugan, G. Kukulka, W. Blue, and A. Roberts. "Effect of Lymphatic and Splenic Pump Techniques on the Antibody Response to Hepatitis B Vaccine: A Pilot Study." *Journal of the American Osteopathic Association* 98 (1998): 155–60.

Johnson, S. M., and M. E. Kurtz. "Conditions and Diagnosis for Which Osteopathic Primary Care Physicians and Specialists Use Osteopathic Manipulative Treatment." *Journal of the American Osteopathic Association* 102 (2002): 527–40.

Jonas, S., and P. Radetsky. *Pace Walking—The Balanced Way to Aerobic Health.* New York: Crown, 1988.

Jones, M. *Growing Old: The Ultimate Freedom.* New York: Human Sciences Press, 1988.

Jones, S. *Darwin's Ghost: The Origin of Species Updated.* New York: Ballantine, 2000.

Journal of the American Osteopathic Association 8 (1908): 3.

Justice, B. *Who Gets Sick: Thinking and Health.* Houston: Peak, 1987.

Kabat-Zinn, J. *Coming to Our Senses.* New York: Hyperion, 2005.

———. *Wherever You Go, There You Are.* New York: Hyperion, 1994.

Kandel, E. R., and F. D. Hawkins. "The Biological Basis of Learning and Individuality." *Scientific American* 267 (1992): 78–86.

Kaptchuk, T., and M. Croucher. *The Healing Arts: Exploring the Medical Ways of the World.* New York: Summit, 1987.

Katie, B., and S. Mitchell. *Loving What Is: Four Questions That Can Change Your Life.* New York: Harmony, 2002.

Keehan, S. P., H. C. Lazenby, M. A. Zezza, and A. C. Catlin. "Age Estimates in the National Health Accounts." *Health Care Financing Review.* http://www.cms.hhs.gov/NationalHealthExpendData/downloads/keehan-age-estimates.pdf (accessed March 20, 2007).

Kenney, R. A. *Physiology of Aging: A Synopsis.* 2nd ed. Chicago: Year Book Medical, 1989.

Kiecolt-Glaser, J. K., L. McGuire, T. F. Robles, and R. Glaser. "Psychoneuroimmunology and Psychosomatic Medicine: Back to the Future." *Psychosomatic Medicine* 64 (2002): 15–28.

Kimberly, P. E. "Formulating a Prescription for Osteopathic Manipulative Treatment." *Journal of the American Osteopathic Association* 79 (1980): 506–13.

———. *Somatic Dysfunction Principles of Manipulative Treatment and Illustrative Procedures for Specific Joint Mobilization.* Kirksville, MO: Kirksville College of Osteopathic Medicine, 1980.

King, H. H., ed. *The Collected Papers of Irvin M. Korr.* Vol. 2. Indianapolis: American Academy of Osteopathy, 1997.

Kinsella, K., and V. A. Velkoff. *An Aging World: 2001.* Washington, DC: US Census Bureau, Series P95/01-1, 2001.

Kline, C. A. "Osteopathic Manipulative Therapy, Antibiotics, and Supportive Therapy in Respiratory Infections in Children: Comparative Study." *Journal of the American Osteopathic Association* 63 (1965): 278–81.

Knebl, J. A., J. H. Shores, R. G. Gamber, W. T. Gray, and K. M. Herron. "Improving Functional Ability in the Elderly via the Spenser Technique, an Osteopathic Manipulative Treatment: A Randomized, Clinical Trial." *Journal of the American Osteopathic Association* 102 (2002): 347–96.

Kobasa, S. C. "Commitment and Coping in Stress Resistance among Lawyers." *Journal of Personality and Social Psychology* 42 (1982): 707–17.

Kobasa, S. C., S. R. Maddi, and S. Courington. "Personality and Constitution as Mediators in the Stress-Illness Relationship." *Journal of Health and Social Behavior* 22 (1981): 368–78.

Kobasa, S. C., S. R. Maddi, and S. Kahn. "Hardiness and Health: A Prospective Study." *Journal of Personality and Social Psychology* 42 (1982): 168–77.

Koop, C. E. "The Health Consequences of Nicotine Addiction: A Report of the Surgeon General." US Department of Health and Human Services, 1988. http://www.cdc.gov/tobacco/sgr/sgr_1988/index.htm (accessed March 1, 2007).

Kornfield, J. *A Path with Heart*. New York: Bantam, 1993.

Korr, I. M. "History of Medicine and the Concept of Endocoids." In *Endocoids*, edited by H. Lal, F. LaBella, and J. Lane. New York: Liss, 1985.

———. "History of Medicine and the Concept of Endocoids." *Progress in Clinical and Biological Research* 192 (1985): 1–4.

———. "Medical Education: The Resistance to Change." *Advances* 4 (1987): 5–10.

———. "Sustained Sympathicotonias as a Factor in Disease." In *The Neurobiologic Mechanisms in Manipulative Therapy*, edited by I. M. Korr. New York: Plenum, 1978.

———, ed. *The Neurobiologic Mechanisms in Manipulative Therapy*. New York: Plenum, 1978.

Kuchera, M., and A. W. Kuchera. *Osteopathic Considerations in Systemic Dysfunction*. Kirksville, MO: Kirksville College of Osteopathic Medicine Press, 1990.

Lal, H., F. LaBella, and J. Lane, eds. *Endocoids*. New York: Liss, 1985.

Larson, E. J. *Evolution*. New York: Random House, 2004.

Leakey, R. *The Origin of Humankind*. New York: Basic Books, 1994.

Lederman, A. "Interview with Maggie Kuhn." *Gray Panther Network* 19 (1990): 3–5.

LeDoux, J. *Synaptic Self: How Our Brains Become Who We Are*. Middlesex, England: Penguin, 2002.

Le Fanu, J. *The Rise and Fall of Modern Medicine*. New York: Carroll and Graf, 1999.

Leuchter, A. F., I. A. Cook, E. A. Witte, M. Morgan, and M. Abrams. "Changes in Brain Function of Depressed Subjects during Treatment with Placebo." *American Journal of Psychiatry* 159 (2002): 122–29.

Leveille, S. G., J. M. Guralnik, L. Ferrucci, and J. A. Langlois. "Aging Successfully until Death in Old Age: Opportunities for Increasing Active Life Expectancy." *American Journal of Epidemiology* 149 (1999): 654–64.

Levkoff, S. E., Y. K. Chee, and S. Noguchi, eds. *Aging in Good Health.* Amherst, NY: Prometheus Books, 2003.

Locke, S., and D. Colligan. *The Healer Within: The New Medicine of Mind & Body.* New York: Mentor, 1986.

Lynch, J. K. "Osteopathic Manipulation Treatment in United States Hospitals: Review of the National Hospital Discharge Survey, 1991–1999." 2000. Abstract.

Maddi, S. R., and S. C. Kobasa. *The Hardy Executive: Health under Stress.* Homewood, IL: Dow Jones-Irwin, 1984.

Marrie, J. T. "Bronchitis and Pneumonia." In *Infectious Disease in the Aging: A Clinical Handbook.* Edited by T. T. Yoshikawa and D. C. Norman. Totowa, NJ: Humana, 2001.

Martin, R. J., B. D. White, and M. G. Hulsey. "The Regulation of Body Weight." *American Scientist* 79 (1991): 528–41.

McGinnis, J. M. "The Tithonus Syndrome: Health and Aging in America." In *Health Promotion and Disease Prevention in the Elderly.* Edited by R. Chernoff and D. A. Lipschitz. New York: Raven, 1988.

McGovern, J. J. "Osteopathically Caring for the Old." *Still University Review* (Fall 2006): 5–6 (repr. from the *German Journal of Osteopathy*).

McGovern, J. J., and R. J. McGovern. "The Evolution of the Mind-Body-Spirit Unit." In *Morphodynamics in Osteopathy*, edited by T. Liem. Hamburg: Hippokrates Thieme Enke, 2006.

———. *Your Healer Within: A Unified Field Theory of Healthcare.* Tucson, AZ: Fenestra, 2003.

McGovern, R. J. "Aging and Osteopathy: The Role of Evidence." *Still University Review* (Fall 2006): 10–13 (repr. from the *German Journal of Osteopathy*).

———, ed. *Special Edition on Osteopathy and Aging Still Review.* Kirksville, MO: A. T. Still University, 2006.

McKeown, T. *The Role of Medicine: Dream, Mirage, or Nemesis?* London: Nuffield Provincial Hospital Trust, 1976.

"Medications and Older People." US Food and Drug Administration. http://www.fda.gov/fdac/features/1997/697_old.html (accessed March 20, 2007).

"Mental Health of the Elderly." American Psychiatric Association. http://healthyminds.org/mentalhealthofelderly.cfm (accessed March 19, 2007).

Millenson, J. R. *Mind Matters.* Seattle: Eastland, 1995.

Mind and Body Special Issue. *Time*, January 29, 2007.

Montgomery, G., and I. Kirsch. "Classical Conditioning and the Placebo Effect." *Pain* 72 (1997): 107–13.

Morbidity and Mortality Weekly Report. "Achievements in Public Health, 1900–1999: Healthier Mothers and Babies." Centers for Disease Control and Prevention, 1999. http://www.cdc.gov/mmwR/preview/mmwrhtml/mm4838a2.htm (accessed March 19, 2007).

Morley, J. E., Z. Glick, and L. Z. Rubenstein. *Geriatric Nutrition: A Comprehensive Review*. 2nd ed. New York: Raven, 1995.

Morley, J. E., and L. van den Berg, eds. *Endocrinology of Aging*. Totowa, NJ: Humana, 1999.

Myers, J., M. Prakash, V. Froelicher, D. Do, S. Partington, and J. F. Atwood. "Exercise Capacity and Mortality among Men Referred for Exercise Testing." *New England Journal of Medicine* 346 (2002): 793–801.

Nathan, B. *Touch and Emotion in Manual Therapy*. New York: Churchill Livingstone, 1999.

National Center for Health Statistics. "Life Expectancy." US Department of Health and Human Services. http://www.cdc.gov/nchs/data/hus/hus06.pdf#027 (accessed March 19, 2007).

National Institute on Aging. "Baltimore Longitudinal Study of Aging." June 10, 2005. http://www.grc.nia.nih.gov/branches/blsa/blsa.htm (accessed March 1, 2007).

———. "Exercise: A Guide from the National Institute on Aging." http://www.niapublications.org/exercisebook/exercisebook.asp (accessed March 26, 2007).

Nelson, M. E. *Strong Women Stay Strong*. New York: Bantam, 1998.

Nesse, R. M., and G. C. Williams. *Why We Get Sick: The New Science of Darwinian Medicine*. New York: Vintage, 1994.

Newman, A. B., A. M. Arnold, B. L. Naydeck, L. P. Fried, G. L. Burke, P. Enright, J. Gottdiener, C. Hirsch, D. O'Leary, and R. Tracy. "'Successful Aging': Effect of Subclinical Cardiovascular Disease." *Archives of Internal Medicine* 163 (2003): 2315–22.

Noll, D. "Osteopathic Manipulation in the Elderly and Current Clinical Research." *Still University Review* (Fall 2006): 14–19 (repr. from the *German Journal of Osteopathy*).

Noll, D. R., B. F. Degenhardt, M. Stuart, R. McGovern, and M. Matteson. "Effectiveness of a Sham Protocol and Adverse Effects in a Clinical Trial of Osteopathic Manipulative Treatment in Nursing Home Patients." *Journal of the American Osteopathic Association* 104 (2004): 107–13.

———. "The Effect of Osteopathic Manipulative Treatment on Immune Response to the Influenza Vaccine in Nursing Home Residents: A Pilot Study." *Alternative Therapies in Health and Medicine* 10, no. 4 (2004): 74–76.

Noll, D. R., and J. C. Johnson. "Revisiting Castlio and Ferris-Swift's Experiments Testing the Effects of Splenic Pump in Normal Individuals." *International Journal of Osteopathic Medicine* 8, no. 4 (2005): 124–30.

Noll, D. R., J. Shores, P. N. Bryman, and E. V. Masterson. "Adjunctive Osteopathic Manipulative Treatment in the Elderly Hospitalized with Pneumonia: A Pilot Study." *Journal of the American Osteopathic Association* 99 (1999): 143–46, 151–52.

———. "Benefits of Osteopathic Manipulative Treatment for Hospitalized Elderly Patients with Pneumonia." *Journal of the American Osteopathic Association* 100 (2000): 776–82.

Noone, G., and W. T. Ang. "The Inferior Boundary Condition of a Continuous Cantilever Beam Model of the Human Spine." *Australasian Physical & Engineering Sciences in Medicine* 19 (1996): 26–30.

Nuland, S. B. *The Wisdom of the Body.* New York: Knopf, 1997.

Ornstein, R. E., and D. Sobel. *The Healing Brain.* New York: Simon and Schuster, 1987.

Paddon-Jones, D., M. Sheffield-Moore, M. G. Cree, S. J. Hewlings, A. Aarsland, R. R. Wolfe, and A. A. Ferrand. "Atrophy and Impaired Muscle Protein Synthesis during Prolonged Inactivity and Stress." *Journal of Clinical Endocrinology and Metabolism* 91 (2006): 4836–41.

Paige, L. *Maybe I'll Pitch Forever.* New York: Doubleday, 2000.

Painter, J. W. "Postural Integration, Transformation of the Whole Self." http://www.bodymindintegration.com/PItransformation.html (accessed March 16, 2007).

Pasteur, L., and J. Lister. *Germ Theory and Its Application to Medicine & on the Antiseptic Principle of the Practice of Surgery.* Amherst, NY: Prometheus Books, 1996.

Patriquin, D. A. "The Evolution of Osteopathic Manipulative Technique: The Spencer Technique." *Journal of the American Osteopathic Association* 92 (1992): 1134–46.

Patterson, M. M. "Research in OMT: What Is the Question and Do We

Understand It?" *Journal of the American Osteopathic Association* 107 (2007): 8–11.

Peel, N. M., R. J. McClure, and H. P. Bartlett. "Behavioral Determinants of Healthy Aging." *American Journal of Preventive Medicine* 28 (2005): 298–304.

Pelletier, K. R. *Mind as Healer, Mind as Slayer: A Holistic Approach to Preventing Stress Disorders.* New York: Delta, 1977.

Pep Up Your Life: A Fitness Book for Seniors. American Association of Retired Persons.

Pert, C. B. *The Molecules of Emotion: The Science Behind Mind-Body Medicine.* New York: Scribner, 1997.

———. "The Wisdom of the Receptors." *Advances* 3 (1986): 8–16.

Peterson, B., ed. *The Collected Papers of Irvin M. Korr.* Colorado Springs, CO: American Academy of Osteopathy, 1979.

Pilisuk, M., and S. H. Parks. *The Healing Web: Social Networks and Human Survival.* Boston: University Press of New England, 1986.

Pope, A. "An Essay on Man." In *Alexander Pope Selected Works*, edited by L. Kronenberger. New York: Modern Library, 1951.

Posinsky, S. H. *Medicine and Anthropology: The New York Academy of Medicine Lectures to the Laity, No. XXI.* Edited by I. Galdston. New York: International Universities Press, 1960.

"Public Resources from ACSM." American College of Sports Medicine. http://www.acsm.org/AM/Template.cfm?Section=General_Public (accessed March 28, 2007).

Ridley, M. *Nature via Nurture: Genes, Experience, and What Makes Us Human.* New York: HarperCollins, 2003.

Rossman, M. L. *Healing Yourself.* New York: Walker, 1987.

Rowe, J. W., and R. L. Kahn. "Human Aging: Usual and Successful." *Science* 237 (1987): 143–49.

———. *Successful Aging.* New York: Pantheon, 1998.

Sagan, L. A. *The Health of Nations.* New York: Basic Books, 1987.

Sandler, H. *Inactivity: Physiological Effects.* Edited by J. Vernikos. New York: Academic Press, 1986.

Sapolsky, R. M. *Why Zebras Don't Get Ulcers.* New York: W. H. Freeman, 1998.

Schiefsky, M. J., trans. *Hippocrates on Ancient Medicine.* New York: Brill, 2005.

Schneider, J. K., A. Eveker, D. R. Bronder, S. E. Meiner, and E. F. Binder.

"Exercise Training Program for Older Adults: Incentives and Disincentives for Participation." *Journal of Gerontological Nursing* 29 (2003): 21–31.

Schwartz, J. M., and S. Begley. *The Mind and the Brain: Neuroplasticity and the Power of Mental Force.* New York: HarperCollins, 2002.

———. *The Mind and the Brain: Neuroplasticity and the Power of Mental Force.* New York: Regan, 2002.

Seeman, T., and X. Chen. "Risk and Protective Factors for Physical Functioning in Older Adults with and without Chronic Conditions: Macarthur Studies of Successful Aging." *Journals of Gerontology, Series B Psychological Sciences and Social Sciences* 57 (2002): S135–S144.

Selkoe, D. J. "Aging Brain, Aging Mind." *Scientific American* 267 (1992): 134–42.

Selye, H. "Stress and Disease." *Science* 122 (1955): 625–31.

———. *The Stress of Life.* New York: McGraw-Hill, 1976.

Siegel, B. S. *Love, Medicine and Miracles.* New York: Harper Row, 1986.

Single, E., D. Collins, B. Easton, H. Harwood, H. Lapsley, P. Kopp, and E. Wilson. *International Guidelines for Estimating the Costs of Substance Abuse.* Ontario, Canada: Canadian Centre on Substance Abuse, 1996.

Social Security Online. "History Archives." 2007. http://www.ssa.gov/history/archives/archives.html (accessed February 28, 2007).

Somers, A. R. "Preventive Health Services for the Elderly: The Growing Consensus." In *Health Promotion and Disease Prevention in the Elderly,* edited by R. Chernoff and D. A. Lipschitz. New York: Raven, 1988.

Spencer, H. "Shoulder Technique." *Journal of the American Osteopathic Association* 15 (1916): 218–20.

Steindler, A. "The Classic: Osteoporosis 1956." *Clinical Orthopaedics and Related Research* 443 (2006): 3–9, discussion 2.

"Steps to a Healthier You." US Department of Agriculture. http://www.mypyramid.gov/ (accessed March 28, 2007).

Sternberg, E. M. *The Balance Within: The Science Connecting Health and Emotions.* New York: W. H. Freeman, 2000.

Still, A. T. *Autobiography of Andrew T. Still.* Kirksville, MO: 1908.

———. *Osteopathy, Research and Practice.* 1910; repr. Seattle: Eastland Press, 1992.

———. *The Philosophy and Mechanical Principles of Osteopathy.* Kansas City, MO: Hudson-Kimberly, 1902.

————. *Philosophy of Osteopathy*. Indianapolis: American Academy of Osteopathy, 1899.

————. *Philosophy of Osteopathy*. Kirksville, MO: 1899.

————. *Research and Practice*. Kirksville, MO: 1910.

Strawbridge, W. J., R. D. Cohen, S. J. Shema, and G. A. Kaplan. "Successful Aging: Predictors and Associated Activities." *American Journal of Epidemiology* 144 (1996): 135–41.

Sugimura, T. "Nutrition and Dietary Carcinogens." *Carcinogenesis* 21 (2000): 387–95.

Syme, S. L. "Psychosocial Interventions to Improve Successful Aging." *Annals of Internal Medicine* 139, no. 5, pt. 2 (2003): 400–402.

Tart, C. *Waking Up*. Boston: Shambhala, 1986.

Thomas, L. *The Fragile Species*. New York: Scribner, 1992.

Toffler, A. *Future Shock*. New York: Bantam, 1971.

Trungpa, C. *Shambhala: The Sacred Path of the Warrior*. Boston: Shambhala, 1988.

Truswell, A. S. "ABC of Nutrition: Some Principles." *British Medical Journal (Clinical Research ed.)* 291 (1985): 1486–90.

US Department of Health and Human Services. "Healthy People 2010." http://www.healthypeople.gov/ (accessed March 23, 2007).

US Food and Drug Administration. "Center for Food Safety & Applied Nutrition." http://www.cfsan.fda.gov/ (accessed March 28, 2007).

US National Institutes of Health. "National Institute on Aging." http://www.nia.nih.gov/ (accessed March 26, 2007).

US Preventive Medicine News. "US Preventive Medicine Introduces Next Generation of Healthcare in America." http://www.uspreventive medicine.com/Press-Room/USPM-News/USPM_Launch.html (accessed March 28, 2007).

US Public Health Service. "Healthy People: The Surgeon General's Report on Health Promotion and Disease Prevention." 1979, http://profiles .nlm.nih.gov/NN/B/B/G/K/ (accessed March 2, 2007).

————. *Promoting Health/Preventing Disease: Objectives for the Nation*. Rockville, MD: US Public Health Service, 1980.

Vita, A. J., R. B. Terry, H. B. Hubert, and J. F. Fries. "Aging, Health Risks, and Cumulative Disability." *New England Journal of Medicine* 338 (1998): 1035–41.

Volpi, E., R. Nazemi, and S. Fujita. "Muscle Tissue Changes with Aging."

Current Opinion in Clinical Nutrition and Metabolic Care 7 (2004): 405–10.

von Faber, M., A. Bootsma-van der Wiel, E. van Exel, J. Gussekloo, A. M. Lagaay, E. van Dongen, D. L. Knook, S. van der Geest, and R. G. Westendorp. "Successful Aging in the Oldest Old: Who Can Be Characterized as Successfully Aged?" *Archives of Internal Medicine* 161 (2001): 2694–2700.

Webster, G. *Sage Sayings of Still*. Los Angeles: Wetzel, 1935.

Weil, A. *Healthy Aging: A Lifelong Guide to Your Physical and Spiritual Well-Being*. New York: Knopf, 2005.

———. *Spontaneous Healing*. New York: Ballantine, 1995.

Weil, A., and R. Daley. *The Healthy Kitchen*. New York: Knopf, 2002.

Wells, M. R., S. Giantinoto, D. D'Agate, R. D. Areman, E. A. Fazzini, D. Dowling, and A. Bosak. "Standard Osteopathic Manipulative Treatment Acutely Improves Gait Performance in Patients with Parkinson's Disease." *Journal of the American Osteopathic Association* 99 (1999): 92–98.

"Whistler, James Abbott McNeill." WebMuseum, Paris. http://www.ibiblio .org/wm/paint/auth/whistler/ (accessed March 28, 2007).

Whitney, E. N., and E. M. N. Hamilton. *Understanding Nutrition*. 2nd ed. St. Paul, MN: West, 1981.

Williams, R. J. "Biochemical Approach to the Study of Personality." *Psychiatric Research Reports* (December 1955): 31–33.

———. *Biochemical Individuality*. New York: Wiley, 1956.

Williams, T. F. "Aging versus Disease." *Generations* (Fall/Winter 1992): 21–25.

Wolff, J. L. "Prevalence, Expenditures, and Complications of Multiple Chronic Conditions in the Elderly." *Archives of Internal Medicine* 162 (2002): 2269–76.

World Health Organization. "About WHO." 2007. http://www.who.int/ about/en/ (accessed February 28, 2007).

INDEX